# The
# Massage
# Bible

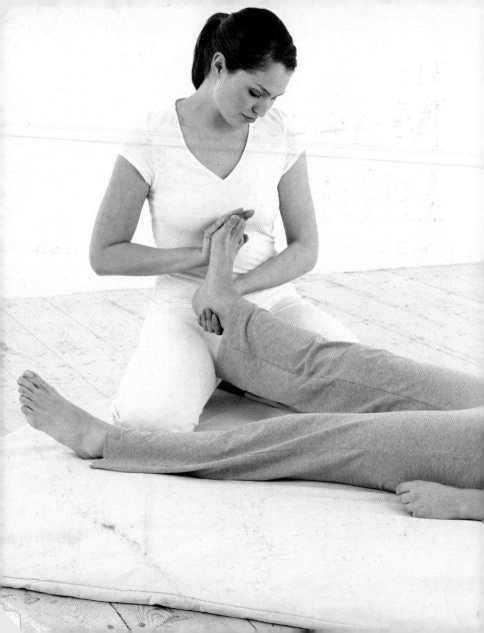

# The
# Massage
# Bible

## The Definitive Guide to Soothing Aches and Pains

Susan Mumford

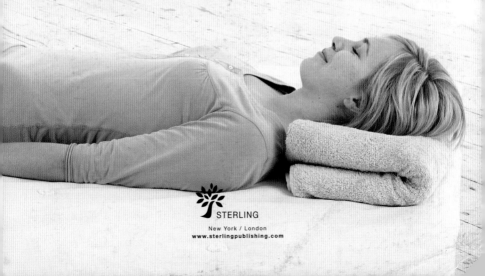

STERLING
New York / London
www.sterlingpublishing.com

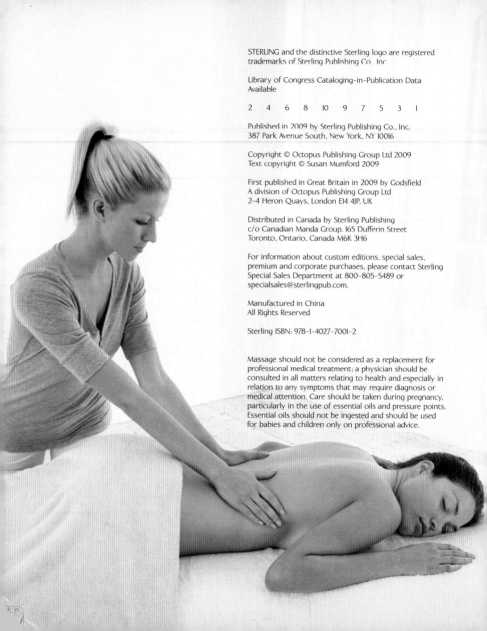

STERLING and the distinctive Sterling logo are registered
trademarks of Sterling Publishing Co., Inc.

Library of Congress Cataloging-in-Publication Data
Available

2   4   6   8   10   9   7   5   3   1

Published in 2009 by Sterling Publishing Co., Inc.
387 Park Avenue South, New York, NY 10016

First published in Great Britain in 2009 by Godsfield
A division of Octopus Publishing Group Ltd
2–4 Heron Quays, London E14 4JP, UK

Distributed in Canada by Sterling Publishing
c/o Canadian Manda Group. 165 Dufferin Street
Toronto, Ontario, Canada M6K 3H6

For information about custom editions, special sales,
premium and corporate purchases, please contact Sterling
Special Sales Department at 800-805-5489 or
specialsales@sterlingpub.com.

Manufactured in China

Sterling ISBN: 978-1-4027-7001-2

Massage should not be considered as a replacement for
professional medical treatment; a physician should be
consulted in all matters relating to health and especially in
relation to any symptoms that may require diagnosis or
medical attention. Care should be taken during pregnancy,
particularly in the use of essential oils and pressure points.
Essential oils should not be ingested and should be used
for babies and children only on professional advice.

# Contents

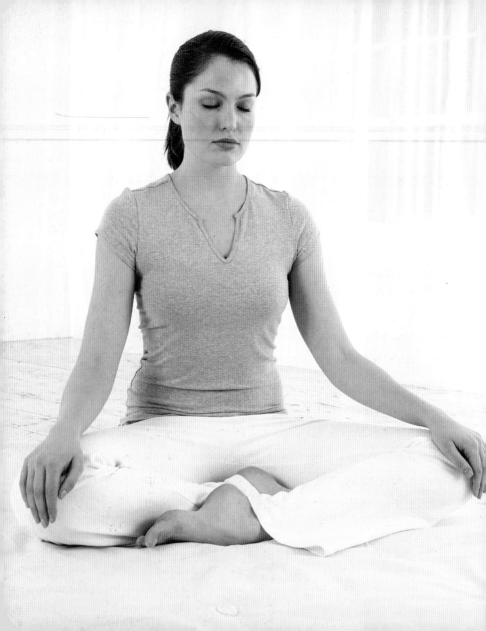

# Introduction

Welcome to this guide, which is going to be a fascinating journey through the world of massage. Massage techniques have evolved over the centuries, incorporating influences from both East and West. As you explore different aspects of massage in this book—from its unrecorded beginnings, through the various techniques and styles, to a step-by-step, full-body massage—you may wish either to dip into certain sections for reference or to follow it all the way through. What will become apparent as you read is how different approaches to massage can complement each other and often overlap. While practitioners often disagree about the best approach, this only serves to keep the art of massage alive and vibrant.

# What is massage?

Massage is basically touch—and touch is something we all do every day. However, while this book will enable you to explore massage and discover your own talent for it, please don't skip straight to the chapter on techniques! Understanding, preparation, and practice are equally important.

Techniques are useful to give structure to a massage, but so are developing empathy and the quality of your touch. It is a question of finding the right balance between them. And once you have mastered the basics and developed your confidence, you can begin adapting your massage to different situations and can even use it to ease everyday common ailments.

## Benefits and styles

A basic understanding of the body provides an insight into the therapeutic benefits of touch. To develop and fine-tune your skills takes discipline and practice. By following each chapter, you will gain a basic understanding of the subject and, with practice and feedback, be able to give a relaxing massage to family and friends. Only a qualified practitioner should offer massage when there are medical problems; if you are in any doubt, always seek medical advice.

Several different massage styles are included in this book. With any style of massage there is one body being treated and two hands doing the treating, which is why the techniques for varying styles have been grouped together loosely—the fundamental difference lies in their approach.

Techniques take time to master and are best practiced first of all on yourself. Look at increasing your flexibility, your mental relaxation, and your sensitivity as a worthwhile investment of your time. All the preparation will finally pay off when the process turns into dynamic interaction with your partner. If you only have a few minutes available for massage, try the quick fixes in each chapter or the self-massage when you are on your own.

*Even if you're short on time, a quick shoulder rub can do wonders to release stress and tension.*

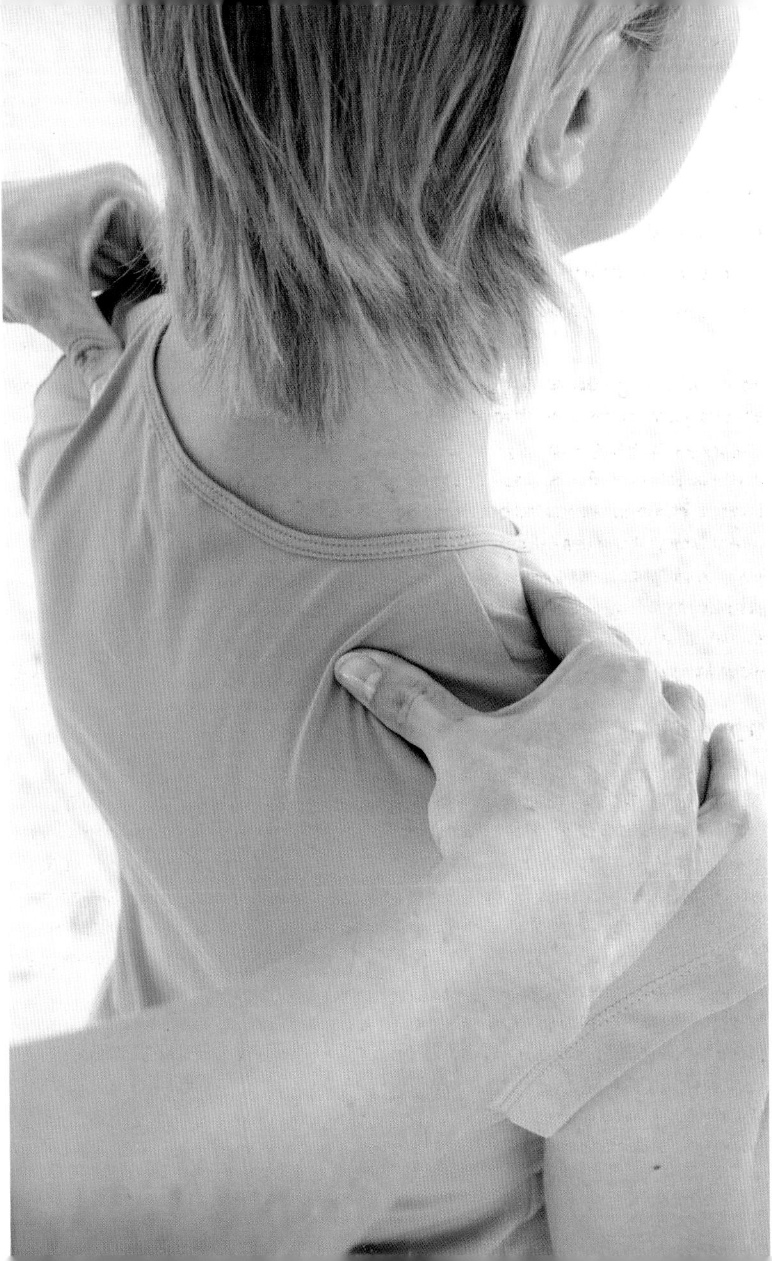

# The history of massage

The origins of massage are timeless. "Rubbing" when things hurt is a natural instinct and is comforting, soothing, and revitalizing. Therapeutic touch is natural to all cultures, so it is difficult to pinpoint its exact beginnings, although various references illustrate the role of massage from past to current times.

## Eastern massage

In China, archeological finds confirm that massage was practiced more than three thousand years ago. The Yellow Emperor's *Treatise of Internal Medicine*, the first comprehensive medical text, compiled sometime between 2700 and 200 BCE, outlined treatment using herbs, acupuncture, and massage. *TuiNa*, meaning "pushing and grasping," sprang from the popular folk massage *anmo*, which survives today. With roots in the Shang Dynasty (starting in 1700 BCE), it emerged in around 1368–1644 CE. In Japan, an early form of massage known as *anma* was introduced from China via Buddhism in the 6th century CE; Western medicine dominated in the early 19th century, but a century later shiatsu emerged and now enjoys official recognition in Japan.

In India, Sanskrit texts dating from around 1500 BCE, forming the basis of Ayurvedic medicine, refer to massage, oils, and herbs. Indian head massage, or champissage (*champi* meaning shampoo), has been part of family grooming for 1,000 years and is used to promote healthy hair. Hieroglyphics found in Egyptian tombs and dated to around 2300 BCE depict practitioners rubbing hands and feet with their hands.

## Western massage

According to Hippocrates, the "father of modern medicine" (c. 460–377 BCE), physicians "should be practiced in many arts but particularly that of rubbing." And the Greek physician Asclepiades of Bithynia (c. 124–40 BCE) recommended massage, diet, exercise, and baths. In Greece, massage was used for digestive ailments and commonly before sport. The Roman physician Celsus (c. 25 BCE– 57 CE) described frictions in detail, recommending massage for headache relief, while Galen (c. 130–201 CE) wrote that "all the muscle fibres should be

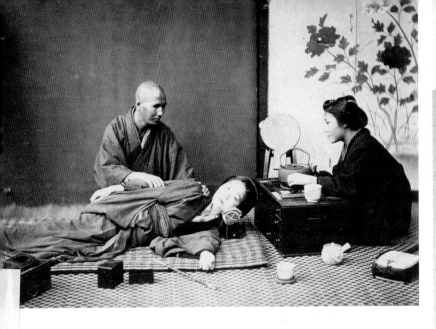

stretched in every direction." Pliny the Elder (23–79 CE) was healed by a medical practitioner of massage, while Julius Caesar (100–44 BCE) received massage for neuralgia. The Persian physician Avicenna (980–1037), who was influenced by Galen, wrote of massage and described various friction methods.

Massage later became frowned upon as indulgent, and medical references are sporadic until the 15th century. In 1813, Per Henrik Ling established the Swedish movement system, although Swedish massage terminology was introduced at a later date by Dutchman Johann Mezger.

*This albumen print from the 19th century, depicts a practitioner attending to a patient in Japan.*

During the First World War injured soldiers were treated with massage, while the Californian bodywork movement of the 1960s combined massage with personal growth.

Each culture has its own traditions, with massage walking a path between pleasure, folk usage, and professional therapy. It is now practiced in its own right, although traditionally it formed part of a therapeutic whole.

# The purpose of massage

Why do we massage, and why is it so popular? Is it done just because it feels nice? It certainly does feel good and a whole health industry has grown up around it, but you could say that the purpose of massage is to benefit both parties that are involved—on many different levels.

## Stress relief

For the purposes of health and well-being, massage stimulates the circulation of the blood, increasing the supply of oxygen to the tissues and lowering blood pressure; it relaxes the muscles and enhances the flexibility of the joints. It also stimulates the nervous system, whether to relax or to increase alertness. Relaxation relieves the effects of stress, which at their worst can cause myriad health problems. In this way massage can be used as a preventative before disease sets in. Stimulation of certain pressure points increases the vitality of the internal organs and can relieve the symptoms of common ailments. Once the body feels at ease, the mind can relax—and switching off may be something that we rarely get to do. The here and now of massage can produce remarkable effects where the stresses of daily life are left behind.

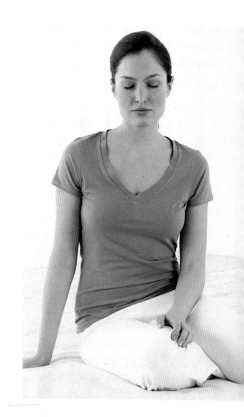

# The healing power of touch

Massage can also be meditative and psychologically healing—for people who may have had a negative experience, massage gives them a chance for positive touch. It is also an acceptable form of touch for those who may not have anyone close to them. It is a way of bonding with a partner, and a wonderful way to bond with a newborn baby. It is a marvelous gift to share and a form of deep communication. It also provides a way of caring and of building confidence that is creative and fun.

Because massage is a great tonic, both physically and emotionally, it helps to improve our appearance. The physical benefits of massage include relaxing tense muscles, which can affect our posture and facial expression; and the boost to the body's circulation improves the color and vitality of our skin. Inner relaxation and feeling good show outwardly in the way we stand and smile.

*The very best massage involves both body and mind which produces a profound state of calm and well-being.*

## CONTRAINDICATIONS

Only massage if you feel energetic and comfortable, and if your partner is in good health. The following physical factors, or contraindications, might make the use of massage inadvisable. Always consult your doctor if in doubt.

Don't massage if your partner has:
▶ an infection
▶ a temperature
▶ heart problems
▶ high blood pressure
▶ untreated cancer

Don't massage over:
▶ varicose veins
▶ an undiagnosed swelling or lumps
▶ skin problems
▶ cuts
▶ a rash

Take care if your partner:
▶ has asthma—always have their medication on hand
▶ is pregnant—pressure must be much lighter; avoid the abdomen during the first four months

Don't massage if you:
▶ are tired
▶ have an infection
▶ are unsure what you are doing

# ANATOMY

A basic understanding of anatomy gives meaning to massage. The body functions as a whole, always working to maintain internal balance, a process known as homeostasis. It is impossible to work on one part of the body without affecting the whole.

# Bones and joints

The underlying structure of the body is the skeleton, which gives the body its shape. It comprises the axial skeleton (made up of the skull, ribs, and spine) and the appendicular skeleton (made up of two girdles: the pectoral girdle at the shoulders and the pelvic girdle at the hips).

Bones are made of living tissue, capable of regeneration. At each end of the bone is a protective cartilage sheath, while in the central shaft is the cell producing bone marrow. Each bone is supplied with blood via its covering of fibrous tissue. Bones protect our vital organs and, in conjunction with the muscles, enable us to move.

## THE BONES OF THE BODY

There are 206 bones in the body, which may be long, short, flat, irregular, or sesamoid (formed in a tendon). The spine, for instance, is made up of 33 vertebrae:

▶ 7 cervical

▶ 12 thoracic

▶ 5 lumbar

▶ 5 sacral

▶ 4 coccygeal

# The ball-and-socket shoulder joint

**Joints** are the meeting point between two bones, enabling us to be flexible. Tendons and ligaments attached to the joint capsule (shoulder or hip) or directly to the bones (knee and elbow) permit movement, while keeping them firmly anchored. Cartilage lying between the bones, as well as sacs of sinovial fluid, acts as a cushion to prevent friction.

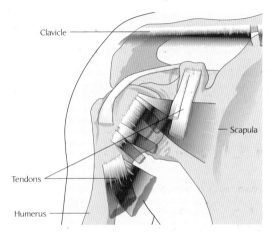

Clavicle

Scapula

Tendons

Humerus

# The hinge knee joint

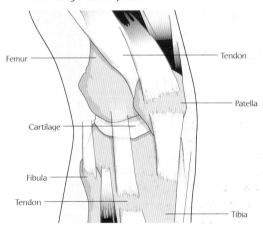

Femur

Tendon

Patella

Cartilage

Fibula

Tendon

Tibia

# Muscles

Skeletal muscles give our body its shape and provide the means for movement. Each muscle is made up of bundles of fibers, which are bound together in a protective sheath. When a muscle contracts in response to a signal from the brain, the fibers slide over one another, shortening the muscle.

The muscle belly is attached to the skeleton by means of tendons at either end, which help to flex or extend the joint. The points at which muscles attach are known as the origin which is the bone the muscle does not move, and the insertion which is the bone it does. Muscles work in pairs or groups, alternately relaxing and contracting to produce movement. Skeletal muscles are under our conscious control and are known as voluntary muscles. Involuntary or smooth muscles, which are not under our conscious control, include the heart and the various organs of digestion.

In order to function properly, muscles require large quantities of nutrients. The blood supplies them with glucose and oxygen, after which it removes the waste products of exertion in the form of lactic acid and urea. Where muscles do not relax sufficiently after working, waste products may remain, slowing the circulation and the uptake of nutrients. This in turn causes stiffness and an increase in resting tone. Over time this may result in the formation of fibrotic tissue—commonly referred to as "knots"—which feel hard and tight and restrict the normal range of movement.

## MASSAGE AND THE MUSCLES

Massage helps the muscles by stimulating normal body processes. Waste products such as lactic acid are released from muscle fibers, enabling the muscles to move more freely. Combined with the benefits of mental relaxation, the increases in muscle tone are returned to an optimum level.

# A guide to the superficial muscles

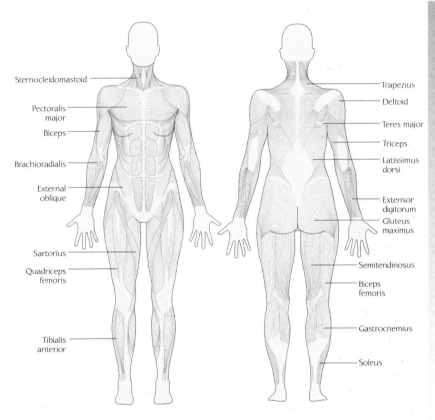

Sternocleidomastoid

Pectoralis major

Biceps

Brachioradialis

External oblique

Sartorius

Quadriceps femoris

Tibialis anterior

Trapezius

Deltoid

Teres major

Triceps

Latissimus dorsi

Extensor digitorum

Gluteus maximus

Semitendinosus

Biceps femoris

Gastrocnemius

Soleus

**The superficial muscles**, as their name suggests, lie nearest to the surface. These muscles are under our conscious control and relax or contract to produce movement.

# The nervous system

The nervous system is our system of communication, both within the body and to our external surroundings. It is essentially our means of interaction with the outside world via stimuli which determine our most appropriate course of action.

The central nervous system is made up of the brain and the spinal cord, and all stimuli must pass through it. Nerves branch off in pairs along the length of the spine, supplying both the limbs and organs. These nerves make up the peripheral nervous system. Spinal nerves supply the body, while those supplying the head are known as cranial nerves. Stimuli pass through the body via sensory receptors in the skin, soft tissue, and muscles. Information is relayed along sensory nerve pathways to the brain via the spinal cord, while impulses from the brain travel back via the motor nerves, enabling us to take appropriate action.

The autonomic nervous system is a complete system in itself. It is concerned with the body's internal processes and is subdivided into two branches: the sympathetic nervous system, which is concerned with speeding up responses, increasing heart rate and breathing; and the parasympathetic nervous system, which slows the body down for repair processes, such as digestion and rest. The body is continually working to maintain a healthy balance between these two systems.

## MASSAGE AND THE NERVOUS SYSTEM

Massage stimulates the central nervous system via the peripheral nerves in the skin. This in turn stimulates the autonomic nervous system. Where overstimulation of one particular system occurs, the therapeutic effects of massage help redress the internal balance, enabling the body to rest and the regenerative processes to take place.

# A guide to the nervous system

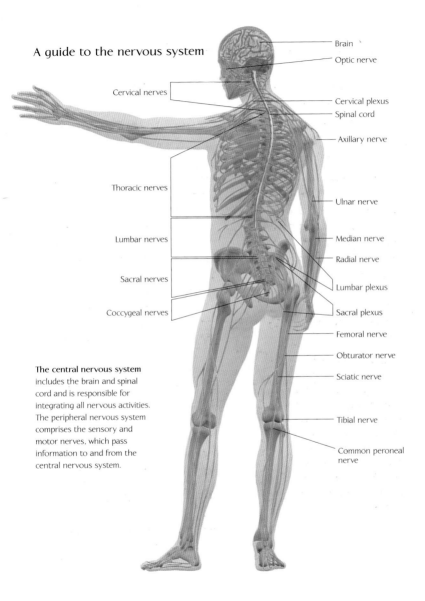

Brain

Optic nerve

Cervical nerves

Cervical plexus

Spinal cord

Axillary nerve

Thoracic nerves

Ulnar nerve

Lumbar nerves

Median nerve

Radial nerve

Sacral nerves

Lumbar plexus

Coccygeal nerves

Sacral plexus

Femoral nerve

Obturator nerve

Sciatic nerve

Tibial nerve

Common peroneal nerve

**The central nervous system** includes the brain and spinal cord and is responsible for integrating all nervous activities. The peripheral nervous system comprises the sensory and motor nerves, which pass information to and from the central nervous system.

# The circulatory system

The blood is the body's transport system, supplying nutrients to the muscles and organs and transporting away metabolic waste. The heart is its major organ; it is a muscle and acts like a pump to circulate blood throughout the body. It has four chambers: two upper atriums and two lower ventricles.

Oxygenated blood is pumped out of the heart via the left ventricle to supply the body through a network of arteries and smaller capillaries, which take nutrients to the tissues. Deoxygenated blood containing carbon dioxide is then transported back toward the heart via the smaller capillaries and veins. The veins in the leg are supplied with valves to aid the flow of blood. Entering the right atrium, the blood is then circulated via the right ventricle to the lungs, where it receives a fresh oxygen supply. It then returns to the heart via the left atrium to begin the journey again.

## BLOOD FACTS

▶ Blood circulates round the body 28 times daily.

▶ It is made up of blood cells (red, white, and platelets) and plasma (nutrients and water).

▶ There are approximately five million red blood cells per 1 ml (0.035 fl oz) of blood.

▶ Red blood cells transport oxygen.

▶ White blood cells fight disease.

▶ Platelets clot the blood.

## MASSAGE AND THE CIRCULATION

Massage helps improve the circulation through stimulation. Waste products are transported from the muscles via capillaries and veins, improving the transport of nutrients to the muscles and organs via the arteries and capillaries. The soothing effects of massage can also have a beneficial effect on heart rate.

# Major blood vessels

The heart acts as a pump for the circulatory system, sending oxygenated blood (shown in red) to the muscles and organs. Deoxygenated blood (shown in blue) is then returned back toward the heart.

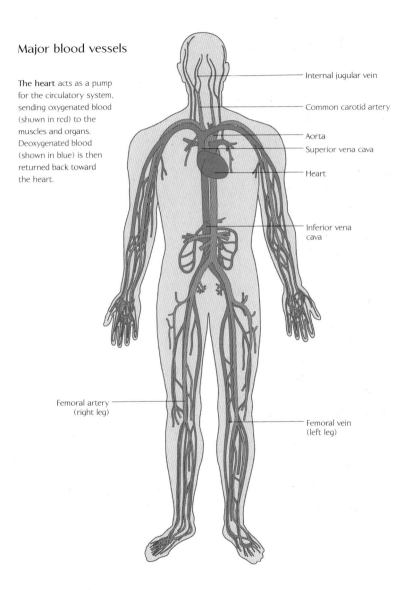

Internal jugular vein

Common carotid artery

Aorta

Superior vena cava

Heart

Inferior vena cava

Femoral artery (right leg)

Femoral vein (left leg)

# The lymphatic system

The lymph system, arising out of the vascular (bloodvessel) system is a means of transport, draining tissues and cells and transporting waste back to the heart via the thoracic and right lymph ducts. It has its own system of vessels: superficial vessels drain the fascia, while deeper vessels drain the organs.

Lymph consists of a clear fluid made up of plasma, fats that are not transported via the veins, proteins, malignant cells, and cell debris. Once it has been collected, tiny valves open and close to transport the lymph. While there is no central muscular pump, skeletal activity and deep breathing assist the flow of lymph. The network of vessels initially takes the lymph toward the nearest lymph nodes for filtration. Lymph nodes are located in clusters at various sites throughout the body, such as the armpits, neck, and groin, and are generally found close to veins. Here waste is processed and sometimes stored, bacteria and unwanted cells are destroyed by immune-system cells known as macrophages, and antibodies are produced by white blood cells known as lymphocytes. The filtered lymph is then returned to the heart.

## MASSAGE AND THE LYMPHATIC SYSTEM

Massage stimulates the removal of metabolic wastes. The lymphatic system is one of the means of transporting these wastes, thus helping to keep the body healthy. Excess fluid or the effects of injury are filtered via the lymph vessels and nodes, helping the body to repair itself and recover from trauma more quickly.

# Lymphatic system

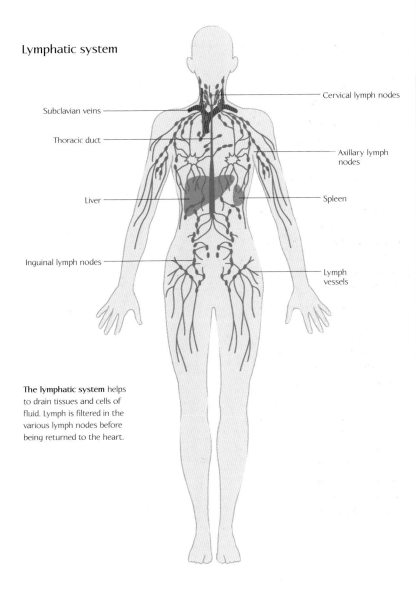

Cervical lymph nodes

Subclavian veins

Thoracic duct

Axillary lymph nodes

Liver

Spleen

Inguinal lymph nodes

Lymph vessels

**The lymphatic system** helps to drain tissues and cells of fluid. Lymph is filtered in the various lymph nodes before being returned to the heart.

# The major organs of the body

The major organs are made of smooth muscle, protected by the ribs and supplied with blood via the circulatory system and nerves that branch out from the spinal cord. Their functions are outside our conscious control and are governed by the autonomic nervous system (see page 18).

## THE ORGANS

| ORGAN | FUNCTION | LOCATION |
| --- | --- | --- |
| Heart | Pumps blood around the body | To the left of center of the chest cavity, between the two lobes of the left lung |
| Lungs | Oxygenate the blood and excrete carbon dioxide | In the chest cavity, protected by the ribs |
| Liver | Breaks down nutrients and cleanses the blood | In the abdominal cavity, over the right dome of the diaphragm, protected by the right lower ribs |
| Stomach | Stores and breaks down food | In the abdominal cavity, over the left dome of the diaphragm, protected by the left lower ribs |
| Kidneys | Maintain fluid balance and excrete waste | At the rear of the abdominal cavity |
| Large intestine | Absorbs water, vitamins, and minerals and eliminates waste | Circles the abdominal cavity, lying around the small intestine |
| Small intestine | Breaks down partially digested food and absorbs nutrients | Connects to the stomach and large intestine |

# A guide to the major organs of the body

**The major organs** of the torso are protected by the ribcage and governed by the autonomic nervous system.

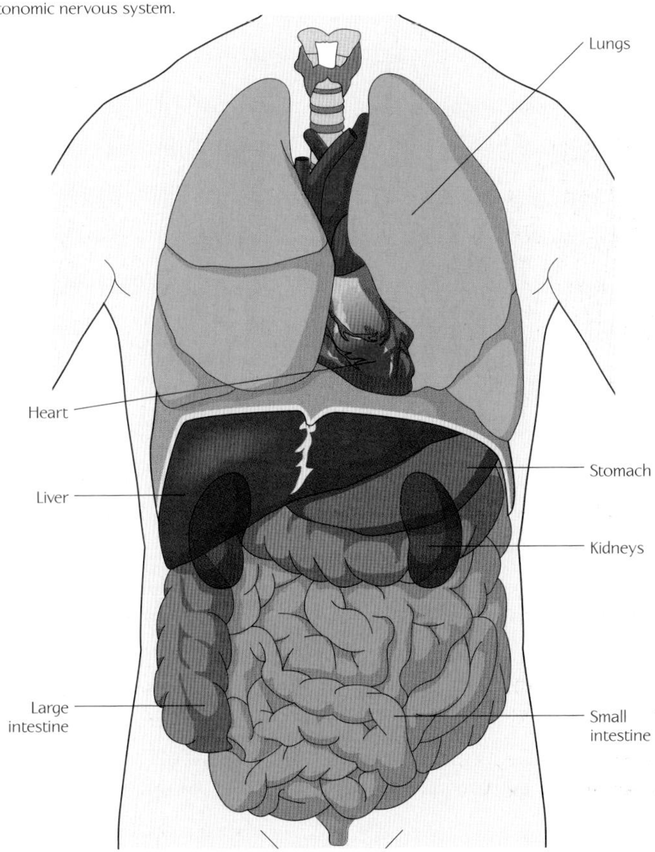

Lungs

Heart

Liver

Large intestine

Stomach

Kidneys

Small intestine

# The skin

The skin is the largest organ of the body, providing our interface with the world around us. It is an organ of excretion, via sweat, which also regulates body temperature. Sensory receptors provide us with immediate feedback about our external environment.

The skin is made up of two major layers: at the base is the dermis (beneath which lies a layer of subcutaneous tissue that supplies nutrients), which is a fibrous layer supplied with blood and lymph vessels, nerves, hair follicles, sweat, and sebaceous glands; above this lies the epidermis, which itself consists of five layers. Dividing cells are continually being produced by the basal layer, and are gradually pushed up toward the outer layer of skin, or corneum. As skin cells reach the surface they gradually die, so that on the surface lie the dead cells that now contain keratin, a fibrous substance that gives the skin its thickness. The skin protects us from bacteria, microrganisms, and harmful influences. Various receptors communicate with the central nervous system and are highly sensitive to touch, pressure, pain, and change in temperature.

## MASSAGE AND THE SKIN

Massage improves the skin by increasing the local blood supply, thus helping to keep it healthy and improving its elasticity. The application of nourishing oils and the friction of the massage strokes also helps to slough off dead surface cells and moisturize the skin at a deeper level.

# The skin

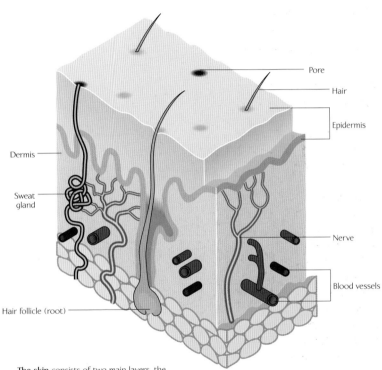

Pore

Hair

Epidermis

Dermis

Sweat gland

Nerve

Blood vessels

Hair follicle (root)

**The skin** consists of two main layers, the upper epidermis and the lower dermis. Rich in sensory nerve endings, the skin is constantly processing information about our surroundings.

# PREPARING FOR MASSAGE

When you're giving a massage it is important to think about the setting. The environment should be restful and inviting, and preparing the room helps to focus your mind, both on the person receiving the treatment and on the reason for massage.

# Setting the environment

You will need a massage table or sufficient floor space; lights that dim; a warm room (the body cools down quickly); peace and quiet, without interruptions; and possibly some background music. A five-minute shoulder rub needs less space than a body massage and can take place almost anywhere, but it is still good to put some thought into it.

Start by creating a soothing environment that makes both of you feel comfortable and relaxed. Candles or oils in a diffuser (see pages 32–33) can add to the ambience for friends and family, but for someone who is less close to you, a clean, uncluttered atmosphere may be more suitable.

It is important to allow enough time: make sure that both you and your partner have allocated plenty of time, not only for the massage, but before and after it as well. Agreeing on a length of time beforehand means that you can both let go and ensure that the massage period is all yours.

## Giving and receiving

Giving a massage is really special. It's something you invest time and energy in for someone else, without asking for anything in return. It's a time when you focus your attention wholly on what you are doing—sometimes that may mean communication without words. While you should attend to your own needs in terms of energy, posture, comfort, abilities, and resources, your attention should primarily be on giving

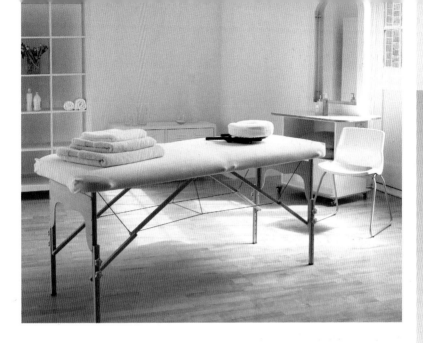

to your partner and being sensitive to their needs and responses. As they respond to the strokes, you may need to adjust your techniques in order for the massage to be a flowing and dynamic experience.

However, nothing much is going to happen if your partner is not open to receiving! The recipient should be encouraged to let you release their tight muscles, rather than holding on to the tension. Their job is to focus on their body and the massage strokes and let you do something for them, without

*The massage environment should be clean and uncluttered yet inviting. Have everything to hand before you start.*

any obligation in return—not as easy as it may sound. Ask your partner to give you feedback throughout and after the massage, in a constructive, non-critical way, remembering that this is a learning experience for both of you. When both participants are focused on the process taking place, then the magic of giving and receiving can be fully appreciated.

# Clothing and equipment

When you are preparing for massage, it is good to have everything you will need ready beforehand and make sure that the massage table is adjusted to your height correctly. That way you can concentrate your mind solely on the massage strokes.

## PREPARATION CHECKLIST

For massage you will need:

▶ A massage table or soft mat on the floor (you can add some padding, if necessary)

▶ A sheet or protective cover to go over the massage surface

▶ At least one large fluffy towel, plus one smaller one for covering the chest area

▶ Oils (see pages 32–33) within easy reach

▶ Supports for the head, knees, or ankles

▶ A glass of water for both giver and receiver

▶ Tissues

▶ Music (optional)

▶ Candles or oils in a diffuser (optional)

Don't forget to:

▶ Remove any jewellery before starting (both giver and receiver)

▶ Tie back long hair

▶ Keep your nails short

▶ Check for any contraindications (see page 13)

▶ Ensure that the room is comfortably warm

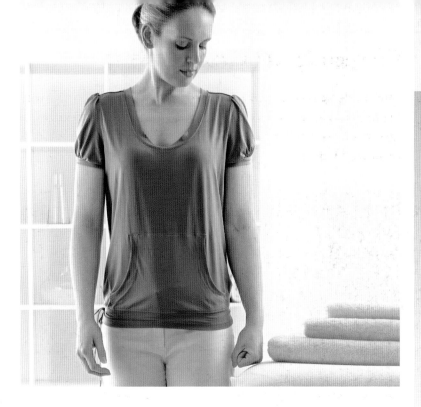

What you wear should be loose and comfortable so that you can bend, stretch, and move freely. You may get oil on your clothes sometimes, so it is best to choose something you can wash easily. For the receiver, clothing depends on what they are most comfortable with: for an oil massage they will need to remove at least some of their clothes (although the body

*Follow the preparation checklist and adjust the table to a comfortable height before you begin your massage.*

areas not being massaged will be covered by towels), but this depends on the massage style: for holistic massage they will have to remove some clothing, but for shiatsu or a head massage they can remain fully clothed.

# Oils and recipes

If you are practicing an oil massage, you will need to have some oil prepared in advance. Its purpose is to help your hands glide over the skin without slipping or sticking. Oils that are used for massage are usually vegetable, nut, or seed oils. Cold-pressed and organic oils from a reputable supplier are best.

## BODY BLENDS

**LIGHT**
Almond 7 ml, Grapeseed 3 ml

**RICH**
Almond 6 ml, Avocado 4 ml
Sunflower 7 ml, Macadamia 3 ml

**NORMAL**
Sunflower 6 ml, Apricot 2 ml,
Jojoba 2 ml

## FACE BLENDS

**SENSITIVE**
Sunflower 4 ml, Jojoba 1 ml

**RICH**
Avocado 4 ml, Macadamia 1 ml

**NORMAL**
Sunflower 3 ml, Rosehip 1 ml,
Apricot 1 ml

Massage also provides an opportunity to nourish and moisturize the skin. Most oils have a shelf life of one to two years and should be stored in a cool, dark place when not in use, to minimize oxidization. New and exotic oils are being introduced regularly. The best policy is to familiarize yourself with a small number at first (such as those given opposite) and then experiment with others as you become more practiced.

## Blend recipes

To prepare an oil blend, make up 2 teaspoons (10 ml) per massage in a glass bottle or bowl; or 1 teaspoon (5 ml) for the face. Allergic reactions are rare, but to be safe, do a patch test on the inside of the elbow and leave for 24 hours. Oil should always be spread over your own hands, rather than applied directly to your partner's skin.

## SUITABLE OILS

| NAME | QUALITIES | HOW TO USE |
| --- | --- | --- |
| Grapeseed oil (*Vitis vinifera*) | A light oil for most skin types | Use as a base or on its own |
| Sweet almond (*Prunus dulcis*) | An all-purpose oil commonly used for massage | Use as a base or on its own |
| Coconut (*Cocos nucifera*) | A heavy, fatty oil that solidifies below room temperature; good for darker skins; long shelf life | Good used on its own for Indian head massage |
| Sunflower (*Helianthus annuus*) | A light, nourishing oil, suitable for children and sensitive skin | Use as a base or on its own |
| Soy bean (*Glycine max*) | An alternative to nut oils, but beware of any sensitivity to this oil | Use on its own |
| Apricot kernel (*Prunus armeniaca*) | A nourishing oil, good for moisturizing the skin, especially the face | Use as part of a blend |
| Avocado (*Persea americana*) | A rich oil for mature skins | Use as part of a blend |
| Macadamia nut (*Macadamia integrifolia*) | A nourishing oil for mature skins | Use as part of a blend |
| Rosehip seed (*Rosa rubiginosa*) | A penetrating, strong-smelling oil, good for wrinkles and scar tissue; short shelf life | Use sparingly as part of a blend |
| Jojoba (*Simmondsia chinensis*) | A silky vegetable wax, good for sensitive skin, especially the face; solidifies below room temperature | Use as part of a blend |

# Posture

Posture is vital when giving a massage, especially if you massage regularly. The natural temptation, especially at the beginning, is to concentrate on getting the strokes right and, in so doing, compromise your own posture. Remember that the massage should be beneficial for both of you.

It is important to use your body weight and make sure that while the massage may come through your hands, the movements are not coming solely from your shoulders. Below are the three main massage postures.

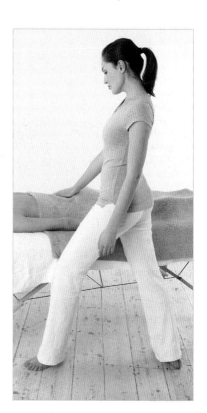

## Working at a table

Make sure both feet are planted shoulder-width on the floor, either side by side or with one foot in front of the other. Keep your spine as straight as possible, bending your knees slightly so that the movement comes from your hips. As you lean forward, your whole body should move without any strain on your neck. Lean your body weight into your hands as you apply pressure, keeping your shoulders relaxed.

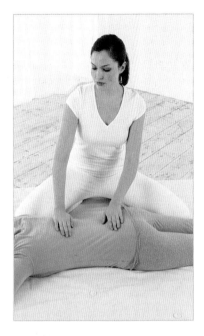

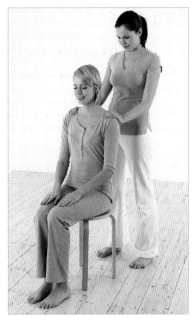

## Working on the floor

Make sure that you are balanced, keeping your knees, ankles, and hips flexible (some padding on the floor is a good idea). Your spine should be straight. To apply pressure, lean forward so that the weight comes through your hips, spine, and shoulders to your hands, with the shoulders remaining relaxed. Apply pressure evenly without overstretching, so that you can regain your original position.

## Working on the head

Stand behind your partner, feet shoulder-width apart and shoulders relaxed. Movement should come from the floor to your shoulders, and through to your arms and hands. Make sure that you do not hunch your shoulders or lean into your partner. To apply pressure, move one foot backward, lean forward through your hips and use your body weight.

# Sensing

Before even starting to massage, it is worth experimenting with the power that naturally comes from your hands. You may be surprised—we all sense our environment and the people in it, often without realizing it. We may brush these feelings aside or be too busy or distracted to listen to them.

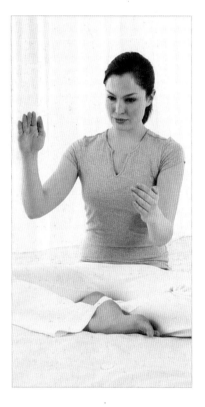

Try these simple exercises to get a sense of the energy coming from your hands. Suspend any preconceptions and experiment to see what you feel.

### Holding an invisible ball

Relax, and rub your hands together until they feel warm. Slowly draw your hands apart, then move them back toward each other. Do this several times and make a note of any sensations that you feel—you may feel a tingling, warmth or that your hands are being drawn toward each other. Try moving your hands around the space as if you are holding an invisible ball, while still keeping a connection between them.

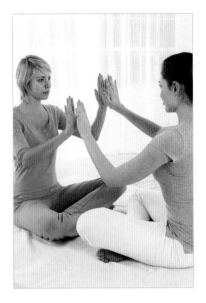

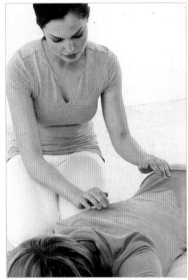

## Establishing a connection

Experiment with a partner. Both of you should hold your hands up, palms facing each other. Keeping a distance between your hands, find the connection between them. Then move your hands to different positions—up, down, backward, and forward—mirroring each other. Notice if the connection changes, and when it feels stronger or weaker. Do all this without actually touching. Notice any sensations or impressions that come through your hands.

## Extending the connection

With your partner lying face down in front of you, hold your hands slightly above their back. Find the distance where you feel that connection without actually touching then. Then see if you can get a sense of your partner simply through your hands. Move them over different areas of the back, again without touching, and see if the sensations change. Then compare impressions with your partner.

# Warm-ups

When you give a massage it is important that you feel relaxed, supple, and alert, so a few exercises to loosen up first are really useful. Wear loose, comfortable clothing and reserve a few minutes for this, so that you can concentrate fully on what you are doing.

## Breathing

Close your eyes. With your shoulders relaxed, take a breath in through your nose. Feel it going right down to your abdomen. As you breathe out, imagine that you are breathing out all the stress and tension from your body. Repeat several times until everything feels looser and you feel calmer mentally.

## Head roll

Lower your chin to your chest and let your head hang. Then slowly roll your head to the left in a big circle, imagining it to be really heavy. When you reach your chest again, circle it the other way. Really *feel* every muscle in your neck moving as you do this. It will help to release any tension.

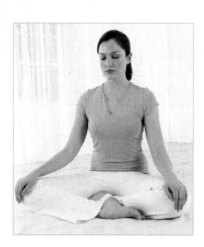

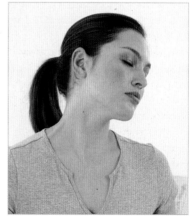

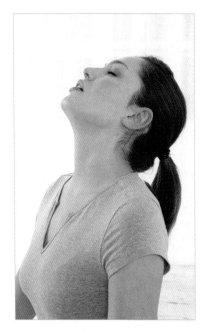

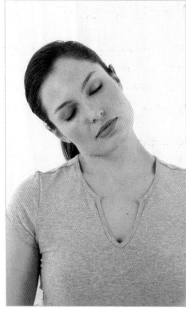

## Backward head tilt

With chin once again on chest, slowly lift your head and continue the movement until you have tilted it back as far as is comfortable. Relax your jaw. Then slowly bring your head up again and take it back once again onto your chest. Then lift it once more, until your head is in the upright position.

## Sideways head tilt

Tilt your head as far as you can toward one shoulder, give an extra stretch and then bring your shoulder up to touch your ear. Bring your head back to a central position and then repeat on the other side.

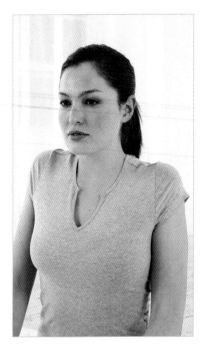

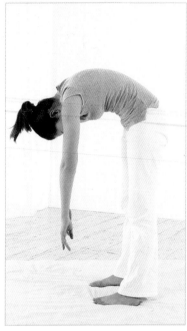

### Shoulder roll

To complete the relaxation of the shoulders, give a huge shrug and bring your shoulders up to your ears. Lower the shoulders, then roll them forward in an exaggerated circle, up to your ears, back and then down. Repeat in the other direction. The muscles should now feel well stretched, relaxed, and much looser.

### Spine roll

Keeping your feet on the ground, flop forward with your knees, neck, and shoulders relaxed. Let your arms and head hang down loosely. Then slowly roll up through the spine, straightening first from your hips. Feel each vertebra as you go, leaving your shoulders and head until last. Once in an upright position, let your head find its natural position of balance.

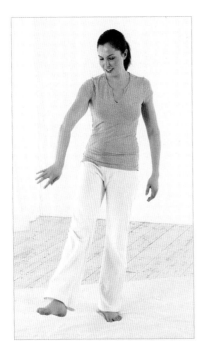

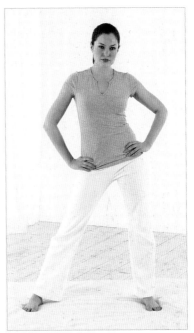

## Shaking out

Now's the time to shake everything out! First, stretch your arms as far as you can to the ceiling, relax them, then shake one arm, followed by the other. All your joints should feel nice and loose. Stand on one leg, and shake the other leg in turn. Concentrate on releasing all the stiffness and tension from your joints.

## Hip circle

With your feet shoulder-width apart, knees slightly bent and hands on your hips, slowly circle your hips to the left. Make an exaggerated circle with them until you come back to your starting position. Then make another generous circle to the right. This helps to loosen the pelvis and lower back.

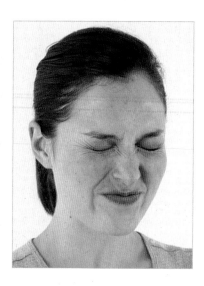

## Face scrunch

To loosen the facial muscles, scrunch your face as tightly as you can. Hold really tensely for a few seconds, then release suddenly, opening your eyes and jaw as wide as possible and sticking your tongue right out! This is really good for waking up your whole system and making you more alert.

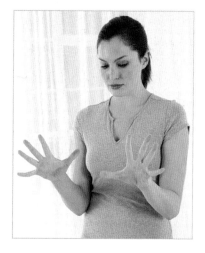

## Finger stretch

To relax your hands, first make really tight fists—as tense as you can—with your fingers tucked right into your palms. Then suddenly release them, straightening the fingers and stretching them as far apart as you can. Repeat energetically several times to exercise the muscles and joints.

## Inward focus

With neck and shoulders relaxed, feet planted shoulder-width apart, and knees slightly bent, focus inward for a few minutes. Concentrate on acquiring a relaxed breath, body and mind. Feel any tension slowly sinking down your body and through the soles of your feet into the ground. You should feel both energized and relaxed.

### THE POWER OF STRETCHING

Stretching and warming up are important to energize your own body before working on someone else. They help to keep you flexible and in tune with your body, and improve your posture and ease of movement. Focus on stretching every muscle, while making sure that you feel relaxed on the inside too. Your concentration should be fully on each exercise in turn. After stretching, make sure you relax every muscle. The more at ease you are with your own body, the more your partner will be able to relax.

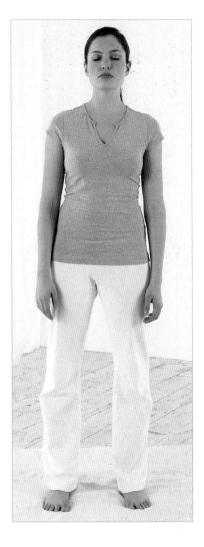

# Sensitivity

When you learn to massage, you can put your sensitivity to good use. Your hands—the main point of contact between you and your partner—are not only the means of performing massage techniques, they also become transmitters: a means of communication between you and your partner.

The palms of your hands are especially important, and relaxed hands and fingers are something you may need to work on, especially when trying out new techniques. Before beginning a massage it is a good idea to sensitize your hands, because this ensures that your attention is flowing in the right direction. So try the following exercises.

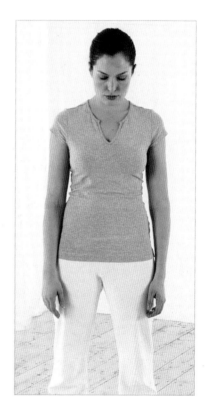

### Feeling the breath
Stand relaxed, with your arms by your sides, feet planted firmly shoulder-width apart on the ground. Take a deep, relaxed breath in and imagine that you are breathing in through the soles of your feet. Feel the breath traveling up through the center of your body to your shoulders. As you exhale, feel the breath traveling down your arms to your hands.

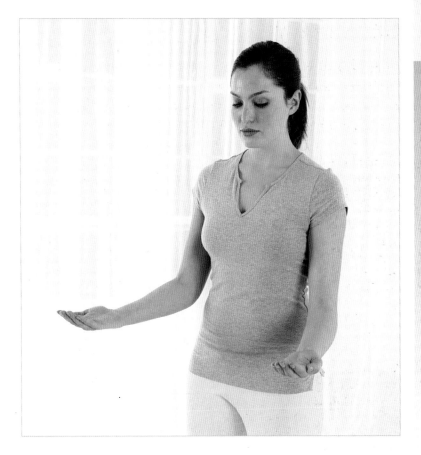

## Energizing the hands

As you breathe into your hands (see opposite), bring your forearms up to the level of your elbows, with the palms facing up. Your hands will feel energized and you may feel tingling sensations in your palms. Repeat the exercise a few times. If you do not feel much at first, don't worry—all these things take a little bit of practice.

# Reading the body

The more massage you do, the more you will start to notice and understand about your partner. The body gives clues as to what is necessary, and you will gain confidence as you learn which areas need attention. You might start to take more notice of the way your partner moves and stands.

Do you see any patterns, or notice any tension? Does anything look uncomfortable or awkward? There are no judgements involved here, just observations, which gradually build up a better picture of how you can help.

Your partner will no doubt point out areas of tension, which are commonly the neck, shoulders, and lower back. And, once you begin to massage, your hands will be feeling for more information. However, when your partner is lying down just before the massage begins, you can take in a great deal of knowledge about them. Here are a few basic pointers to begin with.

1 Neck: Does the head turn easily to the side? If not, this could indicate stiffness.

2 Shoulders: Are they relaxed and lying fairly flat? If not, this could also indicate stiffness.

3 Upper back: Does this look relaxed and fairly flat, or are the shoulder blades very prominent? This may mean that you need to treat the upper back so that the shoulders can relax.

4 Lower back: Is this very arched? It could be placing a strain on the lower back, so this may be an area that you should try and relax.

5 Hips: Are they level? If not, this may indicate lower back or hip problems and an area that could benefit from being relaxed.

6 Hands: Are the hands closed or formed into fists? This may be an area to focus on and a sign that your partner isn't relaxed. If the

joints are painful, massage above and around rather than over them.

7 Legs: Are there any varicose veins? They indicate circulatory problems. You should not massage over the veins themselves.

8 Skin: Does it feel smooth or gritty? Are there any dry patches? This may indicate a lack of hydration and the need to choose a nourishing massage oil.

9 Ankles: Are they puffy? This could mean problems with the circulation or sluggish lymph. Work above, but not over, puffy areas to help drainage.

10 Feet: Is there any redness, or are there any foot problems? Could this be due to wearing tight shoes? Cramped toes really benefit from massage, but do be careful if there are signs of an infection.

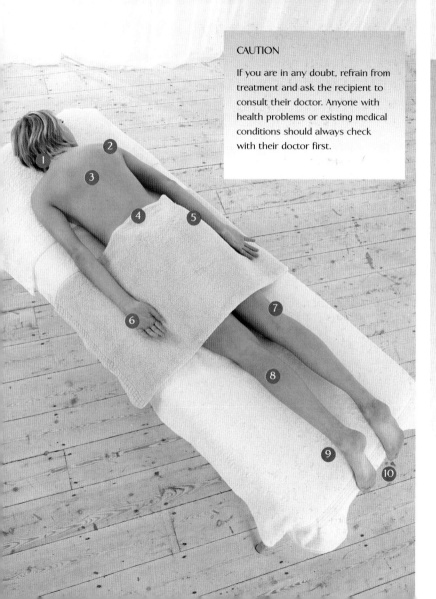

**CAUTION**

If you are in any doubt, refrain from
treatment and ask the recipient to
consult their doctor. Anyone with
health problems or existing medical
conditions should always check
with their doctor first.

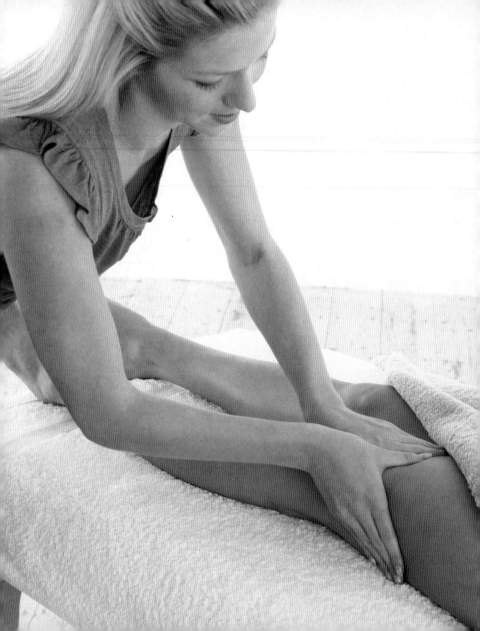

# Techniques

Massage techniques can be broadly divided into light, medium, and deep, traditionally classified as effleurage, petrissage, and friction. For ease of reference the techniques are grouped together here, according to the amount of pressure that is used. Light strokes are used for preparing or closing a sequence; medium strokes help to release muscular tension; and the deeper strokes provide a more focused release. Some techniques are used often, others only from time to time. It helps to familiarize yourself with a few techniques before starting the massage sequences on your partner, and there's no better way than trying them out on yourself.

# How, when, and why

Techniques are something we all want to learn right away! However, massage simply stimulates the body to self-healing, and an understanding of (and interest in) the body and of your partner should come first. Techniques are essential, though: they provide structure and sequence to the massage.

Getting the basic techniques right from the start helps to build confidence in your massage ability and gives you something to practice. You need to balance your techniques and strokes with other factors—a massage based

## TECHNIQUE CHECKLIST

▶ Massage should flow. Make sure that you are in the correct position (see pages 34–35) and physically balanced, so that you can apply the techniques steadily and evenly.

▶ Use relaxing strokes before and after a particular technique to keep the rhythm going.

▶ Start gently, then apply greater pressure as you see how your partner responds. Ease the pressure afterward so that you do not stop abruptly.

▶ Apply the pressure evenly over pressure points, so that you release it just as gradually as you apply it.

▶ Apply techniques appropriate to the area you are working on and the condition you are trying to relieve.

▶ Use techniques appropriate to the muscle groups you are massaging.

▶ Do *not* massage over the spine or bony areas of the body.

▶ Do *not* try to cure any condition with massage techniques.

▶ Use techniques appropriate to your partner's age (less pressure for someone older and less vigorous stretches than for, say, a young person in their twenties).

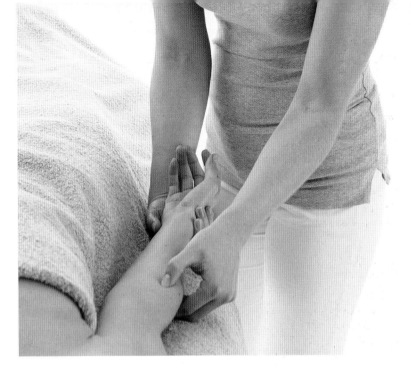

on techniques alone would be a rather empty, clinical affair. So as you practice the techniques, you also need to develop a sense of knowing *why* you are doing what you are doing. Techniques are part of your toolkit. At the outset you will probably follow the routine you have been taught very closely. However, as your knowledge and experience grow, you can be more selective. You don't have to practice every technique every time, and you

*Techniques give structure to your massage sequence. Familiarity comes with practice, giving you a repertoire at your fingertips.*

will gradually learn which techniques are successful in which situations. Developing this ability comes down to practice and experience. The way in which you apply a technique will have an influence on its effect, so bear in mind the balance that you need to achieve every time you massage.

# Pressure

Different massage strokes require different pressures. There are light, flowing, introductory movements over the surface of the skin; medium-pressure, more stimulating movements that may stretch, knead, or roll the tissues; and movements that require deep, very precise pressure over a small surface area.

Gauging pressure is something that you learn by practice and experience and, importantly, through partner feedback. People have very different levels of sensitivity and tolerance to pressure. Some good advice is always to start off lightly and increase the pressure as necessary; varying the pressure gives rhythm and interest to your massage. There needs to be a balance: too light can feel ineffectual and even irritating; too heavy can be painful and make the body tense.

With different techniques and pressures come different contact points of your hands. Some strokes require full-hand contact; others fingers or thumbs; and others just the heels of the hands. These are all part of your massage vocabulary and the fascinating language to be learned.

## Examples of different pressure types

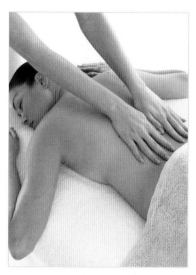

LIGHT PRESSURE:
EFFLEURAGE (SEE PAGE 54)
Long, flowing strokes with soft pressure, using the flat of the hands.

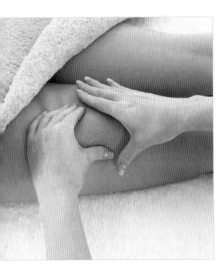

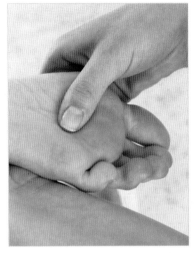

MEDIUM PRESSURE:
KNEADING (SEE PAGE 62)
More robust strokes, applying
stimulating pressure to the muscles,
using principally the fingers and thumbs.

DEEP PRESSURE:
FRICTION (SEE PAGE 82)
Precise pressure into a certain point,
using the fingers or thumb.

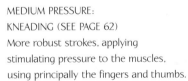

PRESSURE CHECKLIST

▶ Always ask for constructive
   feedback from your partner

▶ Increase the pressure by leaning
   into your hands

▶ Use your body weight, to avoid
   strain on your shoulders

▶ Only use as much pressure as you
   are comfortable with

# LIGHT PRESSURE

Light-pressure techniques should be a soft, comforting introduction to a particular sequence or muscle group. They can be used at any time for reassurance or familiarity during the massage and are important at its close. You can repeat the strokes as often as you like.

# Effleurage

PRESSURE   light
CONTACT   whole hand

Effleurage is a soft, gliding stroke that is often used to spread oil at the beginning of a massage. It is an introduction to your partner's body. The flowing rhythm relaxes the receiver's body and provides an opportunity for the giver to pick up information through their hands. Pressure should be greater when you stroke toward the heart, and lighter on the return.

### How to do it

Rub a little oil over your hands. Then, placing your hands flat on your partner's body at the point nearest to you, and with your hands together, follow the contours of the muscles. Glide as far as you can, then separate your hands and sweep them back lightly toward you. Keep your movements smooth, reassuring, and relaxing.

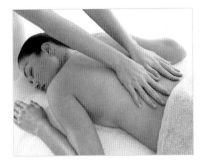

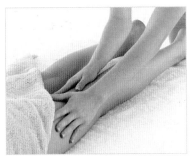

### Effleurage on the back

Position yourself at your partner's head. Spread some oil over your hands and place them at the upper back, just above the level of the shoulder blades. Glide toward the lower back as far as you can reach. Keep full contact between your hands and your partner's body. Separate your hands, reduce the pressure and sweep back up the ribs as you return to your starting position.

### Effleurage on the legs

Position yourself at your partner's feet. Spread some oil over your hands and place them above the ankle. Keep your hands molded to the shape of the leg as you glide up the back of the calf, over the knee, and back of the thigh, as far as you can comfortably reach. Separate your hands and sweep lightly down the outside of the leg to your starting position. The pressure should be reduced over the knee. Avoid any pressure over varicose veins.

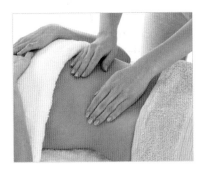

### Effleurage on the abdomen

Place yourself at your partner's side. Spread some oil over your hands and place both hands flat over the abdomen. Then lightly circle them clockwise around the navel, one hand after the other. Keep the pressure fairly light.

# Feathering

PRESSURE  light
CONTACT  fingertips

Feathering is a closing stroke to a massage sequence. It stimulates the surface of the skin and feels reassuring, relaxing, and good. It can draw attention from one area of the body to another, and is a signal that a particular sequence has come to an end. It is mostly used on the back and limbs.

## How to do it
Place your fingertips on your partner's body. Now draw your fingers lightly down the body, a little like stroking a cat. Use your hands in an alternating rhythm so that the movements feel pleasant and smooth. Only one hand is in contact with the body at a time. Gradually lighten and slow your movements down as you near the end of the sequence.

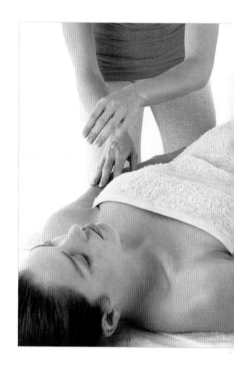

## Feathering the arms
Place your fingertips at the top of your partner's arm. Then softly stroke the length of the arm down to the hand. Use a gentle flowing rhythm, one hand after the other. You can repeat the strokes a number of times and end by lightly stroking over the fingertips.

## Feathering the toes

Cup one hand under your partner's heel for support, and place the other hand at the ankle. Lightly stroke with your fingertips from the ankle to the toes. Repeat several times. Use firmer pressure to avoid the possibility of tickling.

## Feathering the back

Standing at your partner's side, place both hands at the top of the spine (this is one time when you can work over the spine because the pressure is so light). With gentle, alternating movements, lightly brush and stroke down the spine, working your way down to the lower back.

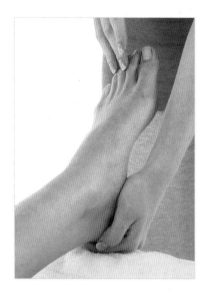

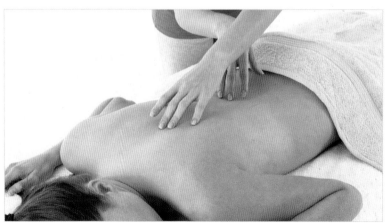

# Rocking

PRESSURE  light
CONTACT  whole hand

Rocking is a good releasing stroke, helping the body to let go of tension. It is helpful as a final release at the end of a sequence, or to relax your partner before the sequence begins. It is a prompt to let go. Rock the limbs or torso with your partner on their back.

## How to do it

Place your hands, with the wrists relaxed and the hands flat, on either side of your partner's body. Push gently in toward the body with one hand, then repeat with your other hand on the opposite side, so that you generate a soft, rocking movement. Change the position of your hands as you rock, so that you move as much of the body as possible. The movements should be gentle and not too fast.

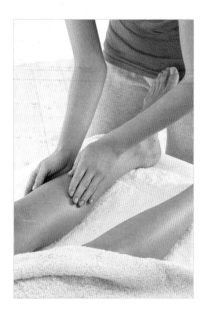

## Rocking the leg

Place your hands on either side of your partner's thigh, facing up the leg. Gently rock the length of the leg, right down to the ankle, using alternate movements with your hands. Repeat back up to the thigh, and end once again at the ankle, making sure that all the joints relax under your hands.

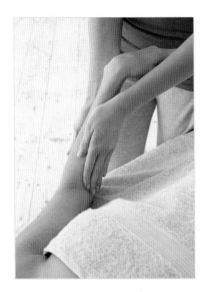

## Rocking the arm

If your partner's arm is supported, you can perform rocking movements with the arm lying flat. Otherwise, lift and place both hands around the upper arm. Without letting go, rock down to the elbow. Bend your partner's arm at the elbow, lowering it to the surface for support, and then continue the movements to the wrist.

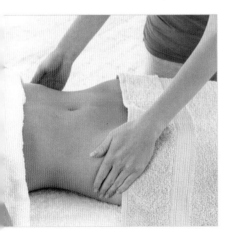

## Rocking the front of the body

Place one hand at your partner's chest and the other at the hips. Begin the rocking movement with your upper hand and follow with the lower. Without disturbing your rhythm, gradually change the position of your hands so that your top hand moves to the hip and your bottom hand moves to the chest.

# Plucking

PRESSURE  light
CONTACT  fingertips and thumbs

Plucking is a light, pleasant, stimulating stroke. Movements alternate between the hands, with the action being staccato and the touch kept light. It is very good for working over the head, or can be substituted for feathering at the end of a body sequence.

## How to do it

Place the fingertips of both hands on your partner's body. Pull one hand away, lightly plucking the surface of the skin as you do so. Repeat the movement with the other hand, alternating your movements to cover the whole area. Keep the movements quick and light.

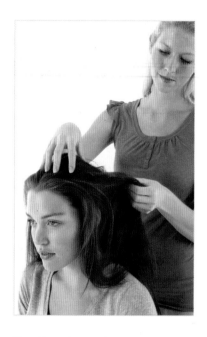

## Plucking the scalp

Stand behind your partner. Place your fingertips on the scalp, then lightly draw one hand away from the head, lightly plucking at the hair as you do so. Repeat the movement with your other hand, alternating with a quick rhythm until you have covered the entire scalp.

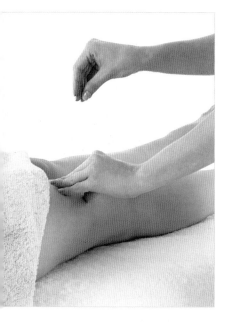

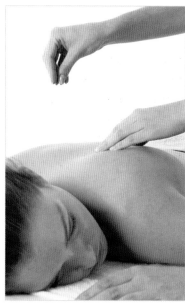

## Plucking the legs

Position yourself at your partner's knee. Place both hands over the thigh and begin the plucking movements away from the body. Work up and down the leg, alternating your hands as you do so. End the sequence at the ankle.

## Plucking the back

At your partner's side, place your hands at the top of the spine. Lightly pluck with your fingertips and thumbs all the way down to the lower back, one hand after the other. This stimulates the surface of the skin and draws the attention down the spine.

# MEDIUM PRESSURE

Medium-pressure techniques help to release tension from the muscles, and are used after oil has been applied with effleurage. Begin the techniques gently; after feedback, you can then increase the pressure until you feel the muscles relax. Apply these to muscular, fleshy areas.

# Kneading

PRESSURE   medium
CONTACT   fingers and thumbs, whole hand

Kneading is one of the more stimulating techniques. Performed after effleurage with oil to prepare the muscles, kneading (as its name suggests) works repetitively over them to relax, release tension, and reduce muscle tone. It is used over larger, fleshy areas, such as the thighs, buttocks, and the muscles on either side of the spine, but is unsuitable for delicate areas or for working over bone.

### How to do it

Place your thumbs and fingertips in position. Press with the thumb, pushing away from you over the muscles; then, without losing contact, grasp the muscles with your fingers and roll back toward your thumb. As you end the movement, begin kneading again in a slightly different position with your other hand, so that you work in a continuous alternating rhythm. Once you have got used to the kneading movements, bring your palms into contact too, for greater effectiveness.

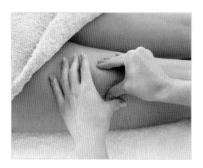

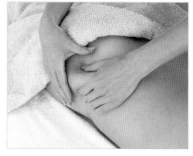

## Kneading the thighs

Position yourself at your partner's side. Press into the muscles with your thumb, rolling back again over the muscles with your fingers. Begin a similar movement with your other hand, alternating the strokes up and down the thigh. Keep to the fleshy muscles, avoiding pressure over the back of the knee and inner thigh.

## Kneading the buttocks

Position yourself at your partner's lower back. Leaning over your partner, begin kneading the opposite buttock, first with one hand and then the other, until you have established a rhythm. Massage over the fleshy areas to release any tension. You can use reasonable pressure, but remember that these muscles can often be quite tender.

## Kneading the back

Position yourself at your partner's back. Lean over and begin kneading the large muscle bands on the opposite side of the spine. Working at least 1 in. (2.5 cm) out from the spine, push your thumbs away from you, then roll your fingers back toward your thumbs. You can work up and down the spine from the lower back to the shoulders, as long as you do not knead over the spine itself.

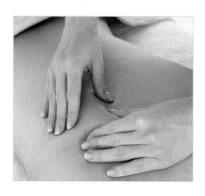

# Squeezing

PRESSURE   medium
CONTACT   whole hand

Squeezing is used upward over the limbs, applying pressure toward the heart. Used after effleurage, it helps to release tension from the muscles as well as stimulate the circulation. The thumbs and forefingers circle the limb while pressure is applied with the whole hand. Squeezing is also good for feeling out "knots."

## How to do it

Place your thumb and forefinger over your partner's limb just above the joint, forming a V shape with your hand. Slowly squeeze up the limb, applying pressure with whole-hand contact. As you move further along the limb, pressure may be applied separately with the hands, spreading them wide to accommodate the body area, without reducing the pressure.

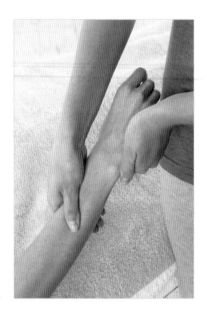

## Squeezing the forearm

Supporting your partner's arm at the wrist, place your thumb and forefinger just above the wrist and squeeze up over the muscles toward the elbow. Contact should now be made with the whole hand. Apply fairly firm pressure, releasing it just below the elbow.

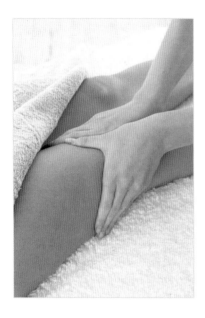

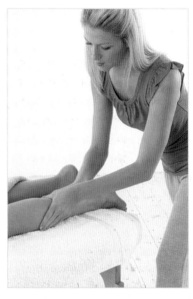

## Squeezing the thigh

Place both hands flat against your partner's thigh, starting just above the knee. With one hand following the other, apply pressure up over the muscles toward the hip. Pressure needs to be fairly firm and the stroke can be repeated several times. Avoid the inner thigh, instead fanning out over the hips.

## Squeezing the calf

Positioning yourself at your partner's feet, place both hands just above the ankle, in a V shape cupping around the leg. Squeeze up toward the knee, applying greatest pressure over the calf muscles. Avoid working over varicose veins, and release the pressure just below the knee.

# Thumb-rolling

PRESSURE   medium
CONTACT   thumbs

Use thumb-rolling to relax muscles, feel out "knots" and connect strokes from one area to another. Use alongside the spine, or over smaller areas like the hands, using the fingers for support. Movements alternate between the thumbs so that you get a continuous rolling effect.

### How to do it

Place one thumb on your partner's body and slowly slide it away from you over the muscles, using medium pressure. As you reach the end of your stroke, lightly lift your thumb off the body to reach your next position. As you do so, begin rolling with the other thumb, so that the strokes alternate and their positions overlap.

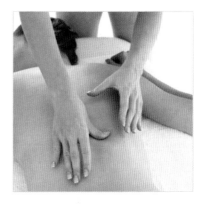

### Thumb-rolling the spine

Position yourself at your partner's head. Leaning forward, begin rolling with one thumb over the muscles to one side of the spine. Alternate with your other thumb, lifting your hands between strokes, right down to the lower back. Repeat several times.

## Thumb-rolling the hand

Supporting your partner's hand with your fingers, use your thumbs to roll over the palm for a good tension release. Roll away from you first with one thumb and then the other, so that you cover as much of the palm as possible. Firm pressure can be effective, but always check the comfort level with your partner.

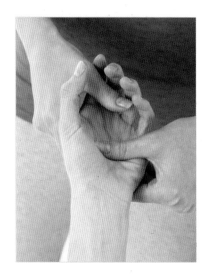

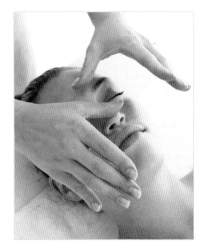

## Thumb-rolling the nose

This is a softer version for working over delicate areas. While working on your partner's face, you can use very gentle thumb-rolling to stroke the length of the nose from the bridge to the tip. Use tiny rolling movements, which feel really comforting, to cover the area.

# Wringing

PRESSURE   medium
CONTACT   whole hand

Wringing is an end-stroke, after working muscles, and may complete a sequence. A good muscle release, it is best used for the limbs or back. It involves a squeezing movement between the hands, but care is needed to oil the muscles adequately so that your hands slide over the skin.

## How to do it

Place one hand on the side of your partner's body nearest to you, and the other on the opposite side. Your hands should be flat against the body and relaxed. Now glide one hand away from you over the muscles, keeping it in constant contact with them. At the same time slide the other hand in the opposite direction back toward you— your hands should meet mid-stroke. Continue until your hands have changed position, then repeat continuously to cover the whole area.

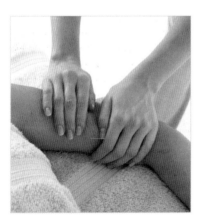

## Wringing the upper arm

Cup both hands around your partner's upper arm. Then slowly wring over the arm toward the wrist, alternating the position of your hands. Keep full contact with your partner's muscles to achieve the wringing effect. Your pressure on the arm should be slightly lighter than elsewhere.

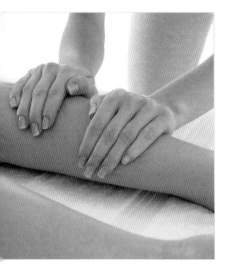

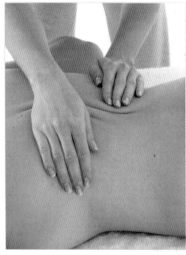

## Wringing the calf

After working over the leg, cup your hands on either side of your partner's calf, starting just below the knee. Pull one hand toward you over the muscles, while sliding the other hand away. Wring down the calf to the ankle. Where the calf muscles are well toned you can use greater pressure, but remember to use plenty of oil.

## Wringing the back

Position yourself square on to your partner's ribs. Mould your nearest hand to your partner's ribcage just below the armpit and, stretching over, place the other hand on the opposite side. Now slide your hands toward each other right over the back, so that they end up on opposite sides. Repeat the movement fairly firmly down to the lower back.

# Circling

PRESSURE   medium
CONTACT   whole hand or thumbs

Circling is for delicate or vulnerable areas and joints. It is a good way to help your partner to relax. Done slowly and rhythmically, with just the right pressure, circling comforts and soothes. Perform whole-hand circles in a counterclockwise direction over the back of the body, and clockwise on the front.

## How to do it
Place both hands flat on your partner's body. Keeping full hand contact, circle over the muscles, with one hand following the other. As you complete the circle with one hand, lift it off gently, making sure the other hand stays in contact with the body. This should be done slowly several times. When using the thumbs only, the principle remains the same, making sure that one thumb always remains in contact with the body.

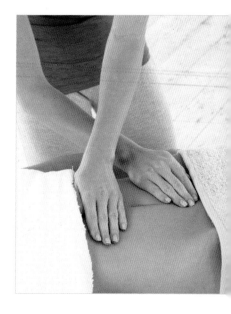

## Circling the abdomen
Position yourself at your partner's side. Place one hand over the abdomen and begin circling clockwise around the navel. Place your other hand on the abdomen to continue the circling movements, lifting one hand lightly when they cross. Use pressure sensitively, and always ensure one hand remains in body contact.

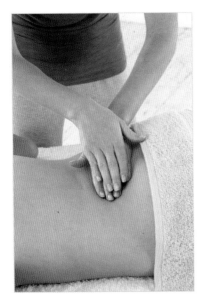

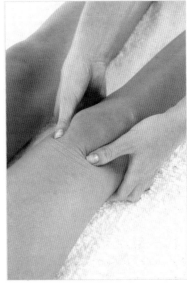

## Circling the lower back

Position yourself at your partner's lower back. Place one hand over the sacrum, the bony area at the base of the spine. With medium pressure, slowly circle your hand counterclockwise, so that it glides over the skin. Use your other hand for support. The more even your pressure, the better it will feel. Repeat several times to ease the lower back.

## Circling the knee

Place one thumb just above your partner's kneecap, and begin circling clockwise around the joint. Join in with your other thumb, circling from the opposite direction. Circle around the joint several times, lifting your thumbs as necessary. This stroke helps the knee joint to relax.

# Palm pressure

PRESSURE   medium
CONTACT   whole hand

Palm pressure is very effective
when used correctly, with your body
weight coming through your hands.
Pressure is applied over the back
and limbs, with or without oil, but
is unsuitable for delicate areas. It
stimulates energy circulation as
well as stretching the tissues.

### How to do it
Make sure your posture is balanced,
then place your hands on your
partner's body. Keeping your hands
flat and relaxed, lean in toward your
partner, using your own weight to
provide the pressure. Apply even
pressure as you perform the movement,
and again as you release. Let the body
respond before changing the position
of your hands.

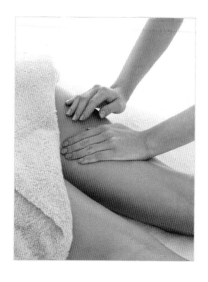

### Palm pressure on the thigh
Position yourself square on to your
partner and place both palms over
the thigh. Use your upper hand as a
support. Lean forward with your weight,
and apply pressure to the muscles with
your lower hand. Continue until you
feel resistance, then release your
pressure slowly and evenly. Pause
before repeating further up the thigh.

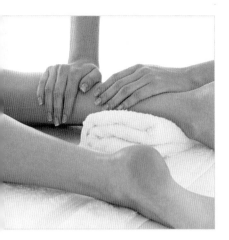

## Palm pressure on the calf

Place a support underneath the ankles. Position yourself square on to your partner and place both your hands over the calf muscles. Lean into the calf with your lower hand, release the pressure, then lean in with your other hand. Move both hands further toward the knee and repeat, but do not press over the joint.

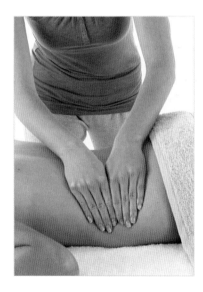

## Palm pressure on the back

Once your partner's back has been massaged, place both hands over the lower back muscles on the opposite side of the spine. Lean into your hands and slide forward, using your body weight. Follow the shape of the body until your hands are curved around the hips. This helps to relax the lower back muscles.

# Rotating

PRESSURE   medium
CONTACT   thumb and fingertips

Rotating stimulates the circulation by applying pressure on the spot over the skin. It is a good releasing and relaxing stroke, working into the muscles as the fingers press. It is not invasive—pressure is distributed evenly by spreading the fingers wide. It is mostly used over the scalp.

## How to do it

Place your fingertips on your partner's body, while raising your wrist and hand. Begin rotating the thumb and fingertips on the spot, applying downward pressure. Keep your fingers in the same position without sliding them over the skin. The movement comes from applying friction to the muscles. After several rotations change position, to cover the whole area.

## Rotating over the head

Standing behind your partner and, supporting the head with one hand, place the fingertips of your other hand on the scalp. Spreading your fingers wide, rotate on the spot and apply pressure toward the scalp. Repeat several times to cover the whole head.

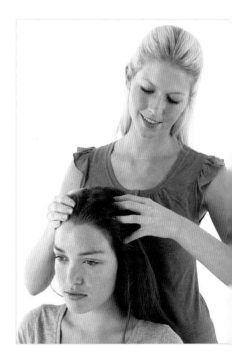

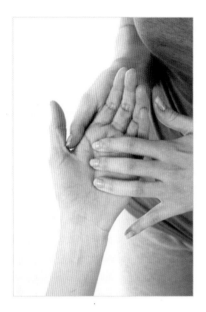
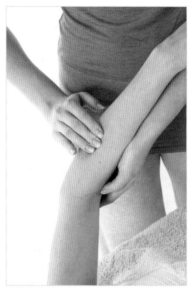

## Rotating over the palm

Support your partner's hand from underneath and place the fingertips of your other hand over the palm. Keeping your wrist and palm raised, rotate in tiny circles over the palm, using the fingertips only. Work over the whole area, applying downward pressure over the muscles.

## Rotating over the forearm

Supporting your partner's arm, place your fingertips on the forearm. Rotate on the spot over the muscles in several positions. The skin should move while your finger contact and pressure remain constant.

# Percussion

PRESSURE   medium
CONTACT   various

Percussion strokes stimulate the circulation through a succession of staccato movements. They should be done quickly over areas of muscle, keeping the fingers and wrists relaxed. They keep body and mind alert and should be used toward the end of a massage sequence.

## How to do it

Keeping the hands, fingers and wrists relaxed, place both your hands on your partner's body. Apply the percussion movements quickly and lightly over the muscles, alternating the strokes between your hands. Cover each area several times, applying pressure more intensely over any tight muscles.

## Cupping

Stand square on to your partner's side. Place both of your hands over the back muscles, with the heels and fingers touching, but leaving space under your palms. Now raise and lower your hands alternately in quick succession, which should produce a hollow "cupping" sound. Work up and down the back, then lean over and repeat on the opposite side of the spine.

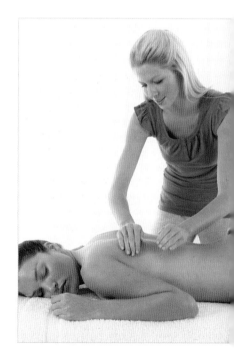

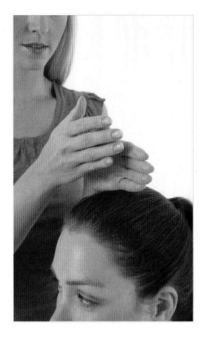

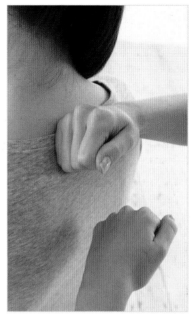

## Hacking

If applied more lightly, percussion can be done on the scalp. Stand behind your partner. Place both hands facing each other on the scalp—contact is made with the little fingers. Now chop your hands alternately up and down, covering the scalp with quick, light movements. The secret is to keep the fingers and wrists loose and relaxed.

## Pummelling

Stand behind your partner, and close your fingers to form loose fists. Place both hands over one shoulder, making contact with the fleshy outer side of the hands. Lightly pummel over the shoulder, moving from the neck out toward the arm. Repeat on the opposite shoulder, then continue up and down on either side of the spine. The more relaxed your wrists, the easier it is to achieve a rhythm.

# Rubbing

PRESSURE  medium
CONTACT  whole hand

Rubbing was the name originally given to massage. This is not a precise stroke, but is used to relax the muscles by vigorous pressure. Rubbing is performed briskly, typically over the scalp or back. Pressure can be applied with the fingers, heel and palm. It is best applied when the skin is not too oily.

## How to do it

Place one hand over your partner's muscles and begin to rub quite vigorously over a small area. Increase the stroke to cover the whole muscle group, applying greater pressure where the muscles feel tight. Keep your hand flat, your wrist loose and perform the movements from side to side.

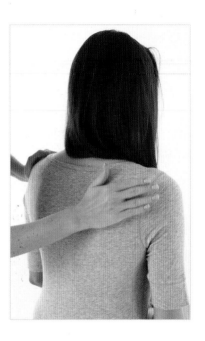

## Rubbing the back

Stand behind your partner. With your hand flat, rub vigorously over the back, avoiding the spine and applying more intense pressure where you feel any tension. The movements should be quick, and both your partner's body and your hands should tingle with the increase in circulation.

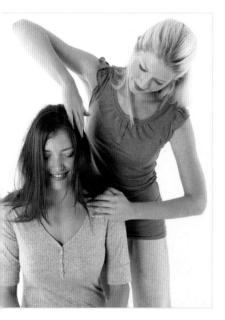

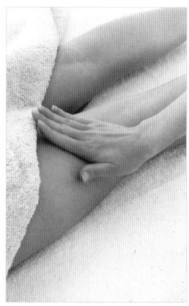

## Rubbing the scalp

Stand behind your partner and begin rubbing lightly over the scalp with one hand, flicking the hair as you do so. Cover the whole scalp with quick, light movements, keeping your wrist and fingers relaxed.

## Rubbing the thigh

Place your hand over your partner's thigh muscles and rub vigorously where they feel tight. This may help at the beginning of a sequence. Rub with side-to-side movements until you can feel some tingling in your palm, helping to prepare the muscles for deeper strokes.

# Stretching with the forearms

PRESSURE  medium
CONTACT  forearms

Forearm stretches are a great
way to relieve tension, providing
pressure with a wonderful sweep.
Applied over muscular areas with oil,
they give a great slide without any
discomfort. Use them as a finishing
stroke, or apply on the spot to
further relax any muscles that
remain tight.

## How to do it

Making sure your posture is balanced
and that you are positioned square on,
lean over your partner and place your
forearms together over the body. Your
hands should be in loose fists and your
wrists relaxed. Now slowly slide your
forearms apart, applying pressure down
toward the body as you do so. Use
your body weight to relax the muscles
and repeat several times, making sure
that no pressure is applied directly over
the bones.

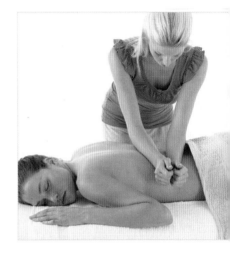

## Stretching over the back

Lean over your partner, with your
forearms facing each other, on the
muscles on the opposite side of the
spine. Apply pressure over the muscles
and, as you do so, slowly rotate your
forearms so that they lie flat against the
body. This is a contained movement and
should be done without too much sliding.
Repeat wherever the muscles are tense.

## Diagonal stretching over the back

Lean over your partner and place your forearms diagonally facing each other on opposite sides of the spine. Slowly draw your arms apart, applying downward pressure and sliding over the muscles, until one arm reaches the shoulder and the other the opposite hip. At the same time, rotate your arms so that the fists and forearms lie flat.

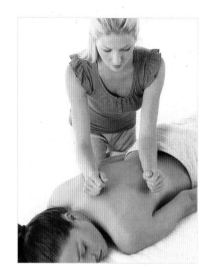

## Stretching over the thigh

Position yourself square on to your partner's thigh. Place your forearms facing each other over the muscles. Slowly draw your arms apart, rotating them as you perform the stroke, until your arms lie flat. Repeat over the thigh muscles, making sure that you complete the movement before reaching the knee or hip. Apply plenty of oil and avoid the inner thigh.

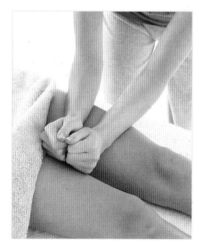

# DEEP PRESSURE

Deep pressure techniques are more focused and release tension from specific areas. They need to be applied carefully to prevent any discomfort. They are intended to be used once or twice, with feedback, and the surrounding area soothed afterward.

# Thumb pressure

PRESSURE  deep
CONTACT  ball of thumb

This is a friction technique whereby pressure is applied precisely over a specific location, typically over a pressure point. This stimulates muscular release, as well as balancing the energy in a particular meridian. Pressure or trigger points are located throughout the body. The movement must be performed with even pressure as well as even release, and must be held for a few moments. The technique is applied after the body has been relaxed.

## How to do it

Locate the point where you are going to apply pressure. Place the ball of your thumb on the surface of your partner's skin, then apply pressure slowly and evenly in toward the body. Focus your attention on the point of contact. Hold for a few moments and then release. Where you feel resistance, relax your pressure, then try again.

### Thumb pressure on the sole

Support your partner's foot in one hand. Locate the point in the center of the foot and hold your thumb over it. Press inward toward the sole, hold for a few moments, then release slowly. Rub very gently over the spot to relax the area and complete the technique.

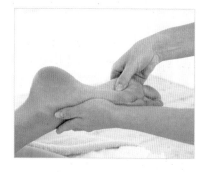

### Thumb pressure on the ankle

Supporting your partner's foot, press right around the joint with your thumb. Press slowly and evenly in toward the joint, and release the pressure equally slowly. This helps to stimulate the circulation and increase mobility. These movements can be followed by passive exercise of the joint.

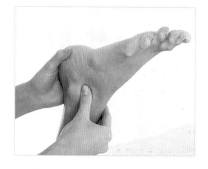

### Thumb pressure on the face

Place both thumbs over your partner's lower eye sockets, the bony ridge just below the eyes. Starting by the bridge of the nose, press in lightly with the thumbs, then release. Continue pressing and releasing at regular intervals, using both hands simultaneously, working along the ridge to the outer corner of the eyes. This helps to refresh the eyes.

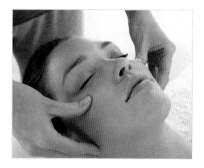

# Finger pressure

PRESSURE   deep
CONTACT   balls of the fingers

Finger pressure is another friction technique, usually performed with two fingers together. It provides less precise pressure over a larger area, which may sometimes be more appropriate. Pressure is applied with the balls of the fingers.

### How to do it
Place your fingertips over the point you are going to stimulate, then press evenly in toward your partner's body with both fingers. Release the pressure slowly. As pressure is distributed between the two digits, the trick is to make sure that you apply the technique evenly between both.

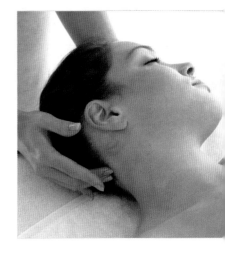

### Finger pressure on the head
Cup your partner's head in one hand, turning it slightly so that you can reach under the skull. Press in with the middle and fourth fingers just beneath the base of the skull, making sure you do not dig in. The muscles there can be quite tight, so this makes a good release. Repeat in several positions.

## Finger pressure on the hip

After working over the thigh muscles, locate your partner's hip joint with your fingertips. Then press into the muscles around the joint with the balls of your fingers. Start gently and release if you feel any resistance, then try again, making sure that your pressure is comfortable and even, but effective.

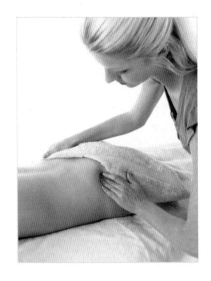

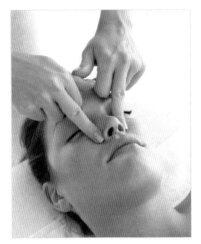

## Finger pressure on the nose

Locate the soft depressions to the side of your partner's nostrils. With steady hands place the middle fingers of both hands over these points, then press gently with your fingertips to stimulate them. The direction is at a slight diagonal in toward the nose. The pressure should be steady, but not too firm.

# Vibration

PRESSURE  deep
CONTACT  balls of the fingers or thumb

Vibration is an extension of thumb and finger pressure. It is used to
stimulate specific points with penetration, so should be used with care.
Avoid the chest or abdomen when working on the front of the body, the
heart area on the back or any painful areas.

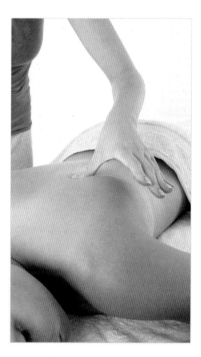

### How to do it
Place your fingers or thumb over the
point you are going to stimulate. Press
in toward your partner's body, but as
you slowly begin to press, vibrate your
thumb or fingers at the same time. This
intensifies the stimulation and you will
find that you can use less pressure.
After a few moments, stop the vibration
and release the pressure as normal.

### Vibration on the back
Locate the relevant point over the
muscles next to your partner's spine.
Place your thumb on the body and
begin pressing into the point, vibrating
your thumb quickly as you do so.
The vibration should be on the spot,
without moving the skin. Release the
pressure slowly without any vibration.

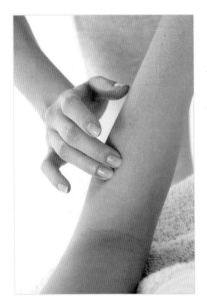

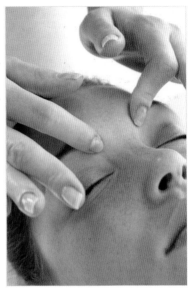

## Vibration on the forearm

Place your middle and fourth fingers over the muscles of your partner's forearm, making sure that you are pressing muscle rather than bone. As you press, begin the vibrating movement with both fingers to increase the penetration. Pause, then release the pressure slowly and evenly.

## Vibration on the face

Place your middle fingers in the bony hollows by your partner's eyebrows. Very, very gently vibrate your fingers on the spot, using hardly any pressure. This technique really helps to energize the eyes and face.

# Heel pressure

PRESSURE   deep
CONTACT   heel of hand

Applying pressure with the heel
of your hand allows you to give
greater depth and pressure to a
stroke. Use it over muscular areas,
putting your body weight behind
the stroke to make it more effective.
This is a robust movement and is
not for delicate or painful areas.

## How to do it
Place your hand on your partner's body
after you have relaxed all the muscles in
that area. Supporting the body against
your pressure with one hand, raise the
palms and fingers of the other hand so
that the only massage contact is with
the heel of your hand. Press downward
and work over the muscles, repeating
the movements several times.

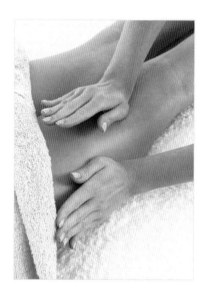

## Heel pressure on the thigh
Standing at your partner's side, place
the heels of both hands over the thigh
muscles. Press in toward the body and
then stroke upward to the hip, with one
hand following the other. You can use
reasonable pressure as long as it is
comfortable. Repeat in several positions,
but avoid the inner thigh.

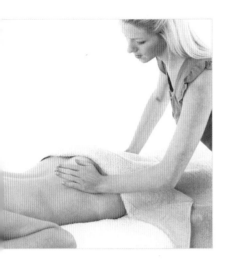

## Heel pressure on the hip

After massaging the lower back and buttocks, press into the muscles around your partner's hip with the heel of your hand and massage around the joint. Support the body with your other hand. Apply pressure firmly into the muscles, circling on the spot for greater release of tension.

## Heel pressure on the head

Use lighter pressure on the head. Stand behind your partner. Supporting the head with one hand, place the heel of your other hand at the base of the skull. Press in toward the muscles, circling and vibrating slightly to increase the stimulation and release. Massage over as much of the area as possible, then complete the treatment by changing hands.

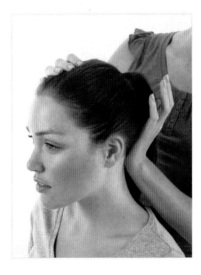

# Knuckle pressure

PRESSURE deep
CONTACT knuckles

Using the knuckles is another way of varying the pressure of your strokes.
It should only be done where the muscles provide some cushioning. It
increases pressure while reducing the stress on your fingers and thumbs.

### How to do it

Placing one hand on your partner's
body for support, make a fist with
your other hand and place it over
the muscles. Gradually increase the
pressure, using your knuckles as the
contact point. Work over the muscles
in several positions, circling over any
tense areas to release them. Varying
the pressure increases your partner's
tolerance to the stroke.

### Knuckle pressure on the hips

After massaging the buttocks, place
your fist over your partner's muscles
and gradually increase the pressure in
toward the body. Circle on the spot as
you press, to increase the stimulation
and encourage the muscles to relax.
Work in several positions, and more
gently around the hip joint, but avoid
any direct pressure on the bones.

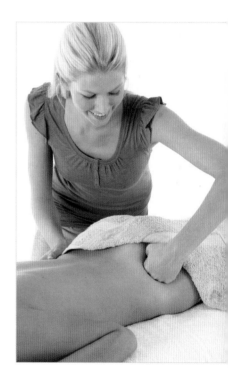

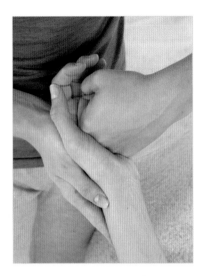

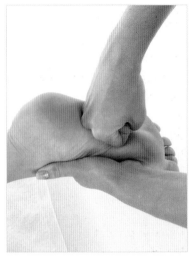

## Knuckle pressure on the palm

Supporting your partner's hand, gently knuckle over the palm, circling in various positions to relax the muscles. Work all around the base of the fingers and thumb, without pressing into the actual joints. Pressure in this way can be surprisingly precise and an effective way of relaxing the hand.

## Knuckle pressure on the sole

Supporting your partner's foot, place your knuckles over the ball of the foot and massage over the soft padding, and then around the base of the toes. Cupping your hand underneath provides resistance against your pressure. Work in small circles on the spot and continue up the outer side of the foot to the heel. Make sure that you avoid putting any pressure over the instep.

# Elbow pressure

PRESSURE  deep
CONTACT  elbow

Using the elbow gives you precise
control over your movements, so
that you can apply pressure
effectively over a muscle or point.
Using your body weight, pressure
is achieved without strain or
compromising your posture. Use
your other hand to steady the
application. Perform carefully,
avoiding delicate areas and bone.

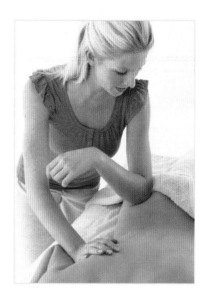

## How to do it
Make sure that your position is
balanced and steady. Position your
elbow touching the part of the body
that you are going to stimulate. Slowly
press into the point with your elbow,
being very sensitive to any resistance.
If your partner resists, ease your
pressure and begin again. Apply the
technique evenly and slowly to help
the body relax.

## Elbow pressure on the hip
Position yourself at your partner's hip.
With your feet planted firmly on the
floor to steady you, locate the relevant
point in the buttock and place your
elbow on the surface of the skin. Slowly
lean into the point with your elbow,
bending your knees to provide balance
and an even pressure. Reinforce the
movement with your other hand,
leaning in slowly and evenly. Release
with equal care.

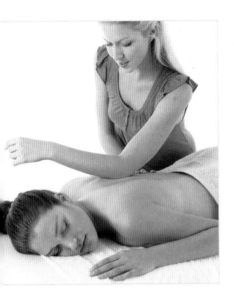

### Elbow pressure on the shoulder blade

Stand behind your partner. Locate the outline of the shoulder blade with one hand, then press around the shoulder blade with your elbow. Guide the movement with your fingers to give precision, and ensure that you don't press directly onto the ribs. Your movements should be small and even, with pressure at a slight diagonal in toward the body.

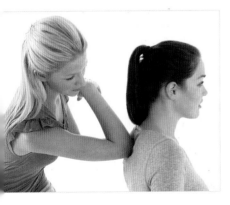

### Elbow pressure on the upper back

After massaging the back, place one finger as a guide over the muscles to the side of your partner's spine. Press gently into the muscles with your elbow, at intervals corresponding to the depressions between the vertebrae. Press once only each time, to the bottom of the ribcage. The pressure should be fairly light and, as always, kept away from the spine.

# Sawing

PRESSURE   deep
CONTACT   fingers and thumb

Sawing achieves depth of movement
and penetration of the muscles. Due
to its effectiveness, it needs careful
application and should only be done
over small areas that are a source
of tension, but not pain. Sawing is
part of your repertoire to apply
after the muscles have relaxed. Use
it selectively.

## How to do it

Place your first two fingers or thumb
on your partner's body. Press down
into the muscle and, as you do so, saw
backward and forward with the fingers
or thumb to intensify the pressure of
your technique. Your fingers should not
slide. You can saw along the length of
the muscle or alternatively across the
muscle belly.

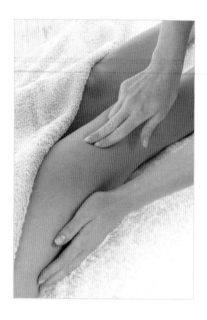

## Sawing the thigh

Place your fingers lengthways over
your partner's thigh muscles. Press
down into them, sawing backward and
forward with your fingers to increase
the penetration. Repeat several times
and then release. Ensure the muscles
are well oiled to prevent uncomfortable
friction with the skin.

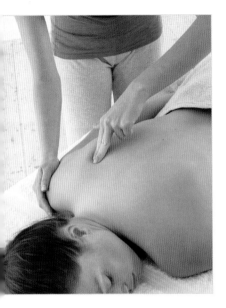

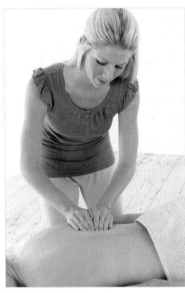

### Sawing the shoulder blade

After massaging around the shoulder blade, begin gently sawing with two fingers wherever your partner's muscles still feel tight. Do this two or three times only, over each spot, before moving on to the next. Continue the movements right around the shoulder blade, but check the comfort levels with your partner.

### Sawing the spine

Stand square on to your partner. If you have already massaged the back, you can focus more attention on particular muscles by applying the sawing technique. Use both hands to saw on the spot over the muscles to the side of the spine. Repeat in several positions over the muscles, but avoid using the technique over the ribs or spine.

# TECHNIQUES FOR THE JOINTS

Techniques for the joints increase the range of movement and flexibility and are used once muscles have relaxed. Work within your partner's range of movement, then extend this slightly by repeating each technique. Feedback from your partner is essential.

# Pulling

Pulling is another name for stretching, and it is great to do after massaging the muscles. It helps to relax the joints, increases mobility, and completes the body sequence. Pulling is a technique for the limbs, but can include the fingers, toes, and neck. Your own position is vital, as is your sensitivity to any resistance. The movements should feel liberating, but should never cause discomfort or pain.

### How to do it

Place both hands around your partner's limb or neck, cupping your hands so that the hold feels comfortable. Slowly pull the body part toward you, so that you feel a slight stretch, then slowly release it again. As you pull, lift the body only as much as is necessary to perform the movement. When you feel resistance you have reached the limit, and you should never try and continue beyond that point.

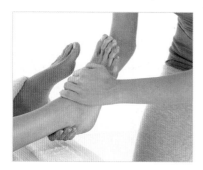

## Pulling the leg

Position yourself at your partner's ankle. Cup one hand over the top of the foot, and the other under the heel. Once your hold is secure, lift the leg slightly and slowly pull the limb toward you. Pull sensitively to the point of resistance, then lower the leg and remove your hands.

## Pulling the neck

Stand at your partner's head. Cup your hands under the base of the skull and lift the head very slightly. Then pull your hands back gently toward you and release. You should notice movement in the upper back. This stretch is very gentle and should last only a few moments, but is very good for helping to relax the neck.

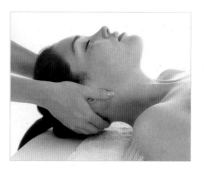

## Pulling the fingers

Support your partner's hand and grasp the tip of one finger between your thumb on the one side and your index and middle finger on the other. Pull toward you to give a good stretch. Repeat with each finger in turn.

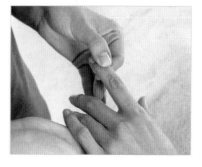

# Passive rotation

Rotating is another way of increasing the flexibility of the joints. A body massage without work on the joints feels incomplete! Encourage and extend the range of movement by applying a little pressure and stretching at the same time. This provides a circulation boost.

## How to do it

Grip with one hand, using the other to steady your partner's body. Now slowly rotate in as big a circle as the joint will permit, applying pressure so that the range of movement increases. Take care that the technique does not cause any pain. Reverse the direction and repeat several times until movement becomes much easier.

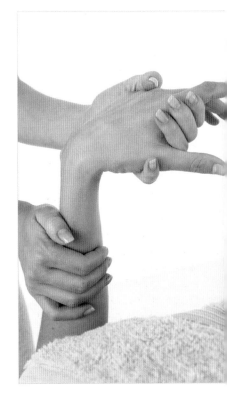

## Passive rotation of the wrist

Supporting your partner's arm at the elbow, grip their hand securely in your own. Keeping the arm steady, begin making a clockwise circle. Make the movement as large as you can, as well as slow and steady. When you have completed the circle, repeat in the opposite direction.

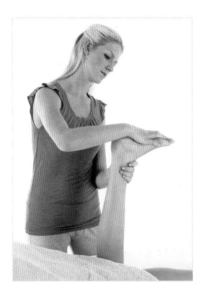

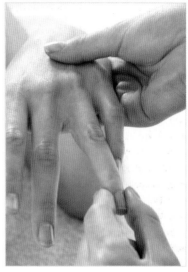

## Passive rotation of the ankle

Support your partner's leg at the ankle. Place one hand flat over the sole of the foot, gripping the ball with your fingers. Slowly rotate the ankle, pressing the foot to extend the movement. Then reverse the direction. The slower you go, the more your partner can simply relax without any resistance.

## Passive rotation of the fingers

Supporting your partner's hand, grasp one finger between your own fingers, pull slightly and gradually rotate it in a big circle. Keep your hands relaxed, and circle each finger in turn, not forgetting the thumb. This small sequence really helps to release tension from the joints by stimulating the circulation.

# Energy-sensing

This is not strictly a massage technique because there is no body contact, but energy-sensing can be used with massage to complete the physical work or to relax beforehand. Your hands should be held in a relaxed position a little away from the body. This technique can be performed over any area.

## How to do it

Breathe into your palms and relax your hands. Now hold them about 2–3 in. (5–8 cm) away from your partner's body. If you feel their body heat, you are getting too close. Hold the same position and imagine that you are breathing out through your hands. Be aware of any sensations or "feedback" that you get from your partner.

## Energy-sensing the lower back

After you have massaged the back area, hold one hand over your partner's lower back, a little away from the spine. Experiment with the distance until it "feels" right. Keep your palm relaxed and just focus your mind on the energy flowing out through your hand. Remain in this position for a few minutes. It will help your partner to relax.

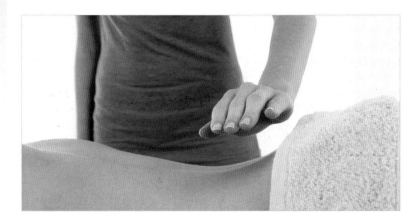

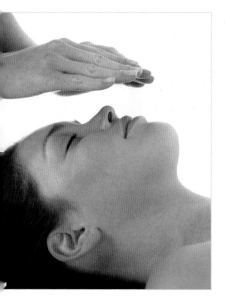

### Energy-sensing the face

After massaging the face, hold both your hands together over your partner's eyes so that they are shaded from any light, but avoid coming too close as this can feel uncomfortable. Imagine that you are breathing out through the palms of your hands. Slowly take your hands away after a few minutes.

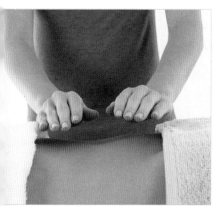

### Energy-sensing the abdomen

After massaging the abdomen, hold both hands still for a moment over it, on either side of the navel. This helps your partner to center. Breathe out through your hands. Wait for your partner to take three full breaths, then gently take your hands away.

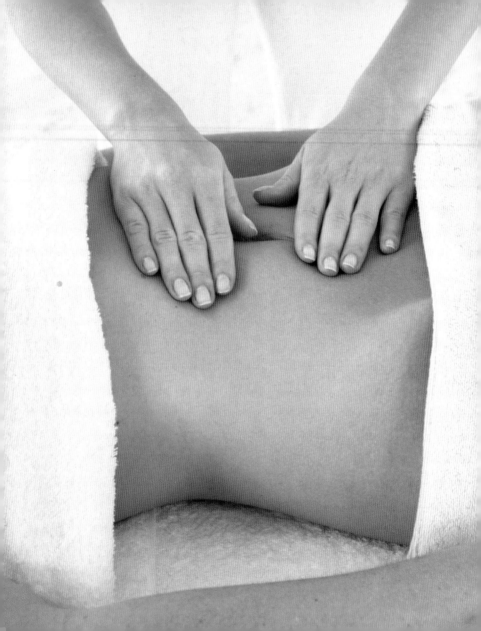

# Holistic massage

The following holistic massage sequence is a mixture
of the techniques that you have just learned (see
pages 48–101). Holistic massage is based on classic
Swedish massage movements, stretches, and a sensitive
interaction with your partner. The rhythm should be
slow and the aim is to relax. The massage combines
gliding movements to spread the oil, firmer strokes to
relax the muscles, and deeper movements to help
release local spots of tension. The massage should feel
like a dance, progressing seamlessly to relax the whole
body. Keep your hands in contact with your partner
wherever possible, and empty your mind of busy
thoughts. Your focus should be on the massage.

# Application

This holistic massage sequence uses techniques that you are now familiar with, in a head-to-toe routine. The massage begins on the back, one of the most important areas for relaxation, offering you a chance to gain confidence with sweeping effleurage strokes.

The massage should move smoothly from one part of the body to the next, following the self-contained routines. The aim is to learn in an interactive process with your partner, rather than give the perfect massage straight off! If some techniques are too difficult for you, come back to them another time, but remember to try and keep your hands moving. Everything gets easier with practice. The massage ends at the feet in order to ground your partner.

## FOCUS POINTS

**Techniques:** The main strokes are effleurage, kneading, squeezing, thumb and finger pressure, and stretching, plus some feel-good strokes such as feathering and rocking (see pages 48–101).

**Movements:** These should be slow and reassuring, moving easily from one stroke to the next. To keep the rhythm, repeat the strokes several times and apply effleurage rather than stopping.

**Equipment:** You need a firm surface such as a massage table or soft mat on the floor; towels to cover the body areas you are not working on; supports for the head, knees, or ankles; and some oil (see pages 30–33).

**Feedback:** Make a note of any problem areas before you start and always ask your partner for feedback.

**Timing:** A body massage takes about 45 minutes; a back massage about 20 minutes.

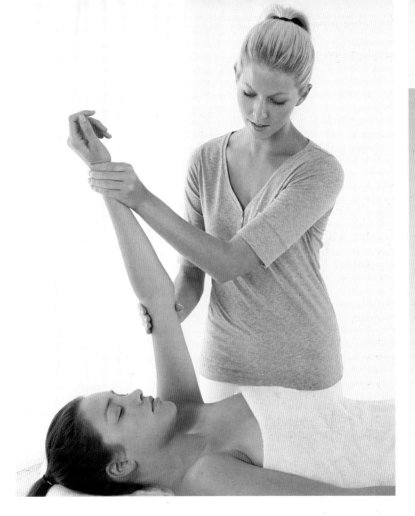

*Explore the massage sequence with your
partner as part of a dynamic learning
process. Keep movements flowing.*

# The back

This is the beginning of your massage, so make sure that you have to hand everything you will need and center yourself first. Then enjoy the long, sweeping stokes down the length of the back and the chance to massage some large muscle groups.

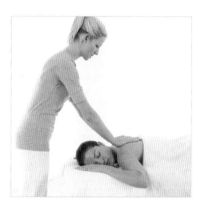

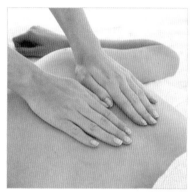

1 first touch Position yourself at your partner's head (see Posture on pages 34–35). Check that your partner is comfortable. Empty your mind, breathe slowly, and relax. Focus on your body, and imagine that you are breathing in through your feet and slowly out through your hands. As you exhale, place your hands flat on your partner's back and relax for a few moments. This sets the tone for the massage.

2 effleurage Rub a little oil between your hands. Lean forward, placing your palms together flat on the upper back. Sweep as far down toward the lower back as you can. Your hands should lie flat against your partner's body in continuous contact and should mould themselves to your partner's muscles. Effleurage spreads the oil, relaxes your partner and is an opportunity to feel for any tension.

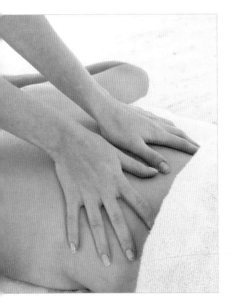

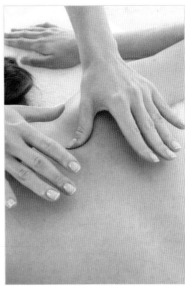

3 effleurage As you reach the end of your downward stroke, spread your fingers and separate your hands so that they return up either side of the ribcage. Pressure should be lighter on the upward stroke. Come back to your starting position and repeat the movements several times. Your hands should glide and feel reassuring, without using too much pressure.

4 thumb-rolling Place both thumbs on the muscles to the side of the spine, in the triangle between the neck and the shoulder blade. Roll with the balls of your thumbs in continuous movements down the side of the spine. The pressure should be enough to relax the muscles, but not painful. Check the pressure with your partner before repeating.

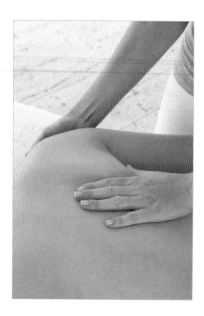

5 palm pressure Support the shoulder with one hand underneath, and place the palm of the other hand flat on your partner's upper back, with the fingers curled over the top of the shoulder. Draw your hand around the outline of the shoulder blade, applying pressure down toward the body. Repeat several times to relax the muscles, pressing as close in to the shoulder blade as you can.

6 thumb pressure Still supporting with the lower hand, press in with your thumb around the shoulder blade, pressing between (but not directly on) the ribs. Press evenly with the ball of your thumb, hold for a moment each time and then release. This stimulates the muscles between the ribs, as well as helping the shoulder to relax.

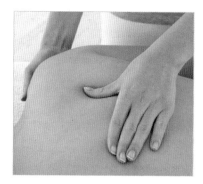

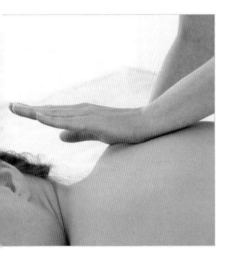

7 heel pressure Still supporting the shoulder, place the heel of your hand over the shoulder blade itself. Apply pressure as you move diagonally over the muscles, releasing it as you massage toward the arm. Press and circle with your heel where the muscles feel tight, with your other hand providing cushioned resistance.

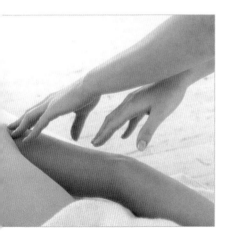

8 feathering To end the sequence, lightly feather with both fingertips down the length of your partner's arm. Brush lightly, drawing the focus away from the back to the hand. Repeat several times, then move back to the head and begin the entire sequence on the other side. Always work with the head turned away from the shoulder that you are massaging.

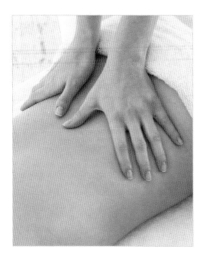

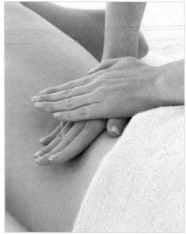

9 effleurage Move to your partner's
lower back and rub some oil between
your hands. Place your palms together
over the sacrum, the triangle of bone
at the base of the spine. Spread your
fingers and separate your hands so
that they sweep up and out over the
lower back and hips. Return to the
starting position and repeat with
pressure on the outward sweep.

10 circling Position yourself square
on to your partner. Place your hands
flat over the sacrum, with one on
top of the other to steady the
movement. Apply a little pressure
with your upper hand and begin
making a counterclockwise circle.
Repeat very slowly and evenly to relax
the lower back without any discomfort,
keeping your hands flexible and molded
to the body.

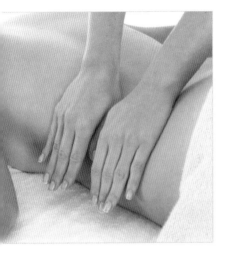

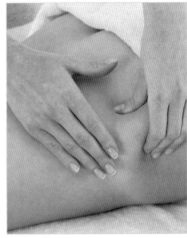

11 **palm pressure** Place your hands together on the lower back muscles on the opposite side of the spine. Apply pressure with the palms of your hands, as you roll away from you over the muscles and sweep around the hip to the buttock. The contact should become lighter and change to the fingertips as you complete the stroke.

12 **kneading** Leaning over, begin kneading the buttock. Press into the muscles and roll the flesh back toward your thumbs with your fingers, so that you achieve a rhythmic rolling movement. Your hands should alternate. Continue massaging with a fairly firm pressure on the muscles only until they feel relaxed.

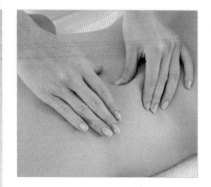

13 kneading Continue the movement by kneading the muscles on the opposite side of your partner's spine, pressing in with your thumbs and rolling back toward you with your fingers. Avoid working over the spine itself—allow roughly 1 in. (2.5 cm) either side of it. Massage up to the shoulder and back down again, then change position and repeat the lower back sequence on the other side.

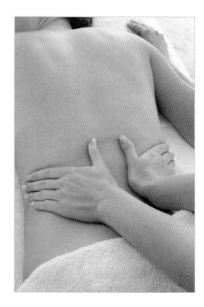

14 palm pressure Place the heels of your hands facing away from each other at either side of the lower back. Slide your hands in opposite directions out toward the ribcage, using full hand contact toward the end of the stroke. Repeat at intervals until you reach the shoulders, where you should just apply pressure between the shoulder blades.

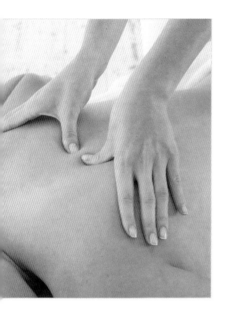

15 thumb pressure Beginning between the shoulder blades, place both thumbs over the muscles on either side of the spine. Press in simultaneously with the balls of the thumbs, pressing at intervals parallel to each vertebra. Press firmly but sensitively; never press into the bone. Move quickly and evenly down to the lower back.

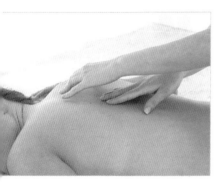

16 feathering To end the back sequence, place your fingertips once again at the top of the spine and lightly feather down to the lower back. Repeat in alternating, rolling strokes to draw awareness down the body. Rest both hands on the lower back for a moment, then lightly withdraw your touch.

# Back of the legs and feet

Position yourself where you can massage the length of the legs and complete each sequence on one side of the body before beginning on the other side. Aim to use similar pressure on both sides. This is a great opportunity to work on the joints after relaxing the muscles.

1 **effleurage** Position yourself at your partner's feet. Spread some oil over your hands and place them together just above the ankle. Glide with your hands together over the calf, reducing the pressure at the knee, and continuing the stroke to the hip. Separate your hands at the top of the thigh and return more lightly down the outside of the leg to the ankle.

2 **squeezing** Wrap your hands around the leg just below the calf. Create a V shape between your thumbs and forefingers and grip lightly with your fingers. Squeeze up over the calf toward the knee, where you should lighten the pressure and end the stroke. Repeat, but do not massage over any varicose veins.

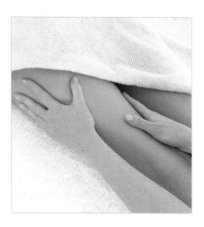

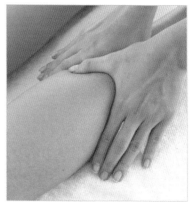

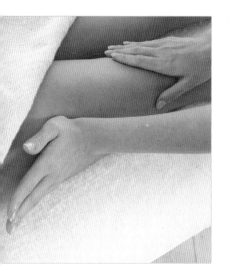

3 heel pressure Continue the squeezing stroke up the thigh, then use the heels of your hands for more pressure. These muscles tend to be quite toned, so you can safely use your body weight. Avoid the inner thigh. Keep your hands at an angle so that there is no contact with your fingers or palms.

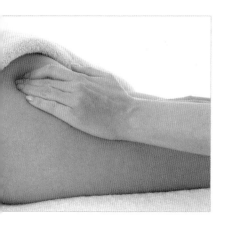

4 finger pressure Use the balls of your fingers to press around the hip joint. Once you have located the joint, press in around it with your middle and fourth fingers, applying pressure evenly in and releasing evenly out again. Check with your partner because this area can be sensitive, but the muscular release feels very good.

5 kneading Adjust your position to stand square on to your partner. Place your hands over the thigh muscles and knead, pressing in with one thumb and rolling your fingers back toward you, as you do so beginning the stroke with the other hand. Knead over the muscles to relax them, avoiding pressure on the inner thigh and knee.

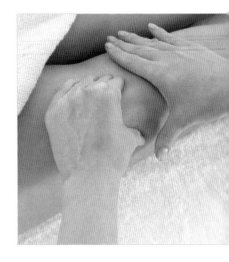

6 wringing Place your hands at either side of the lower leg, just below the knee. Wring over the leg with both hands—one sliding toward and the other away from you. Continue quickly and lightly toward the ankle, keeping full hand contact. Make sure that you slide, rather than pulling the skin, and apply more oil if necessary.

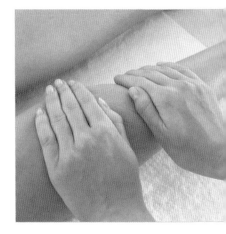

7 rotating Bend the lower leg back and support it at the ankle with one hand, while the other hand grasps the sole of the foot. Your fingers should be over the ball, with the palm firmly over the sole. Begin slowly rotating the ankle, taking it through its full range of movement. Repeat the movement in the opposite direction, then slowly lower the leg back down.

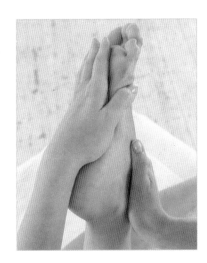

8 pulling Place one hand underneath the ankle, and the other just above the heel. Lift the leg slightly with your lower hand and pull it gently toward you. You may notice the effect in the hip. Your partner should relax the leg without trying to straighten it or help. Release your hold gently and stroke over the foot.

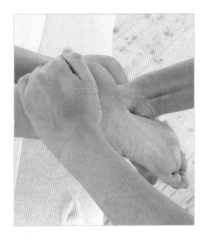

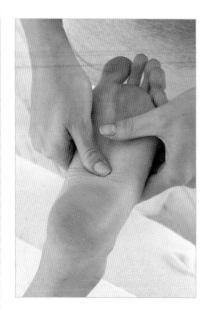

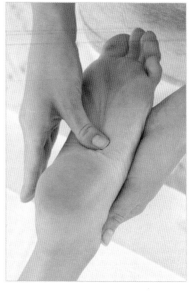

9 **thumb-rolling** Massaging the feet ends the leg sequence and makes it feel complete. Support your partner's foot from underneath and use your thumbs to roll over the soles of the feet. Pressure should come from the balls of your thumbs. Begin movements in the middle of the foot and slide toward the sides. Cover the whole area, excluding the instep, several times with alternating, rolling movements.

10 **thumb pressure** To further relax the foot, press over the sole with your thumb, making tiny circles on the spot. Keep the movements continuous and pay particular attention to pressing in around the base of the toes and over the ball of the foot. Your pressure can be quite firm, but be aware of any spots that might be tender to the touch.

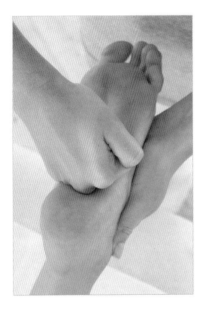

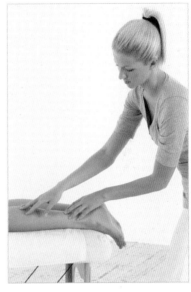

11 knuckle pressure Cushioning the foot from underneath, press down over the sole with your knuckles, making small circles on the spot. Keep the pressure comfortable and avoid working over the instep. Check for comfort and any tenderness as you work. Gently lower the foot and stroke over it with your fingertips.

12 feathering Brush with your fingertips from the hip to the toes with long, light, flowing movements. Keep enough hand contact to avoid tickling. Relaxed, loose wrists will help your movements, drawing your partner's focus right down to the feet. Slow your strokes as you end, then change position and repeat the entire sequence on the other leg.

# The neck and scalp

Work on the front of the body should be a little more gentle than that on the back. Most people have neck tension and find it hard to let go, so work within your partner's limits. Stretches provide great release. The more confident your touch, the better your movements will feel.

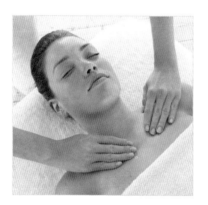

1 effleurage Rub the smallest quantity of oil over your fingers. Positioned at your partner's head, place your hands on either shoulder, then sweep around over the shoulders until your hands meet at the back of the neck. Draw your hands up slowly to the base of the skull and release. Repeat several times to give your partner confidence and to aid relaxation.

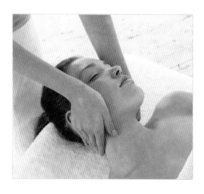

2 rocking This is a very slow, gentle, sensitive movement designed to relax the neck. Place one hand on one side of your partner's neck, just below the skull. Full contact should be made with your palm. Gently rock to one side, guiding the movement with your hand. As the head turns to the side, begin a second rocking movement with the other palm, so that the head turns back the other way. Repeat several times.

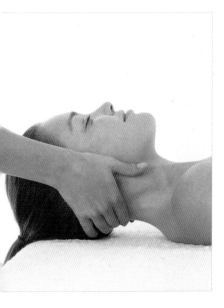

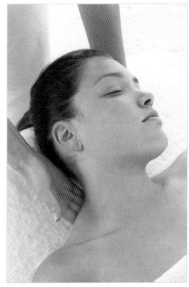

3 **pulling** Place your hands together
under the neck, and cup the base of
the skull. Lift the head slightly and pull
it very gently toward you, then release
and lower the head slowly. This gives a
good stretch, but must be avoided if
there are any neck problems. This
technique takes practice and is best
done with your partner's feedback to
help you.

4 **finger pressure** Turn the head by
cupping your fingers around your
partner's ears and supporting it with
both hands. Rest the head on one hand
while you reach under the opposite
shoulder with the other. Draw up your
fingers along the muscles to the side
of the spine, pressing toward the body
until you reach the base of the skull.

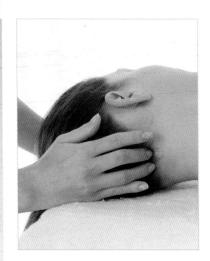

5 finger pressure Press around the base of your partner's skull with your fingers, starting to the side of the spine and moving toward the ear. The pressure should be right beneath the skull, but not too deep as this area can be very sensitive. Press slowly and evenly for the best results.

6 palm pressure Place the palm of your hand over the top of your partner's shoulder. Maintain full contact and slowly draw it over the muscles, sweeping up toward neck. End the movement at the base of the skull. Keep your hand moulded to the body for a luxurious, relaxing stroke. Repeat several times.

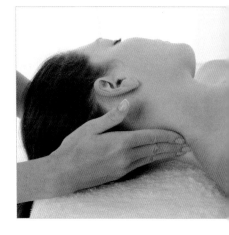

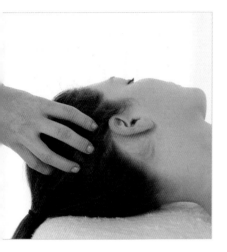

7 rotating From the base of the skull, move your fingertips just above the hairline and begin small rotations on the spot over the scalp, covering as much of the head as you can reach. The pressure can be fairly firm, but take care not to tug the hair. Then change hands and repeat the neck sequence on the other side.

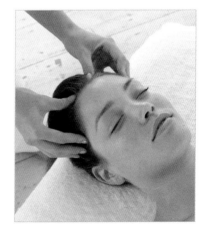

8 rotating With the head back in the central position, place both your hands over the front of the scalp and rotate on the spot, a bit like shampooing the hair. Then draw your fingers through the hair to end the movements and thoroughly relax your partner.

# The face

Face massage feels blissful. The skin on the face is delicate, so you need to keep your hands steady, your movements precise, and your strokes soft, especially around the eye area. Pressure can be firmer when working on male skin, especially around the jaw.

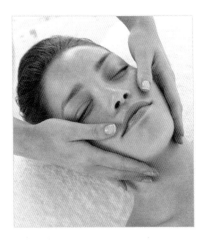

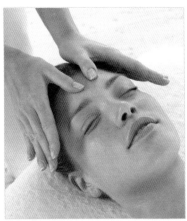

1 effleurage Rub a small quantity of oil between your fingers. Lightly spread it over your partner's skin by applying three sweeping strokes outward over the face, covering the forehead, cheeks, and chin. Lift your hands to avoid the eyes, and only apply sufficient oil to enable your fingers to glide.

2 thumb pressure Place the length of your thumbs together in the middle of the forehead. Slowly draw them outward to the temples in a sweeping stroke. Repeat in roughly three lines until you have covered the area, the last stroke being just above the eyebrows. This is good for mental as well as physical relaxation.

3 thumb pressure Place the tips of
your thumbs on each eyebrow, just
beside the bridge of the nose. Draw
them out over the eyebrows toward
the temples, then release. You can
apply a reasonable amount of pressure.
Contact should be made with the sides
of your thumbs. Repeat several times to
relax the brow and eyes.

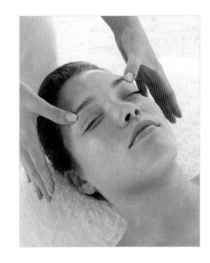

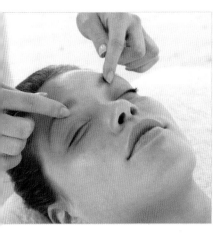

4 finger and thumb pressure
Place the tips of your index fingers just
below the eyebrows on the bony ridges
of the eye sockets. Using both hands
simultaneously, press lightly at even
intervals toward the outer corner of
the eyes. To work along the lower
ridge, change to pressure with your
thumbs, repeating the small movements
along the sockets back toward the
bridge of the nose.

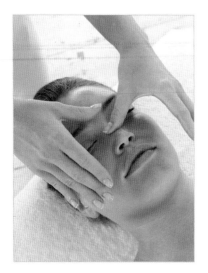

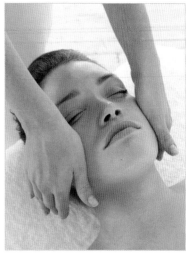

5 **thumb-rolling** Place both thumbs just below the bridge of your partner's nose and then apply small, light, rolling movements down to the tip. Work with your thumbs at a slight angle and keep your fingers raised so that they don't brush the face or, more especially, make contact with the eyes. Use the strokes alternately to bring your hands into position to massage over the cheeks.

6 **heel pressure** Place both hands at a slight diagonal above the face, with the heels of the hands on either side of the nose. When you have got the right position, make contact and sweep out over the cheekbones with your heels. Some pressure over the cheeks feels fine, but gradually reduce it as you reach the ears. Repeat several times, making sure that you have enough oil not to stretch the skin.

7 heel pressure Now repeat the
stroke, starting at the chin and
sweeping out over the lower jaw. Keep
your hands molded to the shape of the
jaw and sweep up toward the ears. Lift
your hands gently at the end of the
stroke and repeat several times. You can
also make use of your fingers and palms.

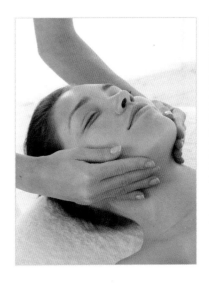

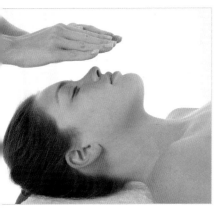

8 energy-sensing Place both your
hands slightly above your partner's
face, with the palms roughly covering
the eyes. Just rest and calm your mind.
Focus your attention on your hands
and any sensations that you feel,
without changing your position. Then
focus on your partner's face and again
note any sensations. Lift your hands
away gently to complete the sequence.

# The arms and hands

This sequence provides a chance to release the shoulder area and massage the hands, which always feels wonderful. Massage one side of the body first, then the other, and use similar pressure on each arm. The inner arms can be quite sensitive, so less pressure is needed here.

1 effleurage Rub some oil between your hands and position yourself at your partner's side. Place both hands just above the wrist and sweep up over the arm toward the shoulder. At the shoulder your hands should separate and brush back down more lightly to the wrist. This stroke helps you to apply the oil and prepares the arm for massage.

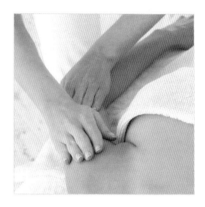

2 squeezing Supporting the arm with one hand, place your fingers and thumb just above the wrist and squeeze up over the forearm toward the elbow. Apply pressure with the web of your hand between the thumb and index finger. Ease the pressure toward the elbow and repeat, moving your hand to a slightly different position each time.

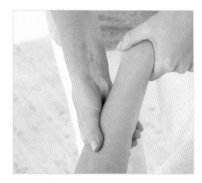

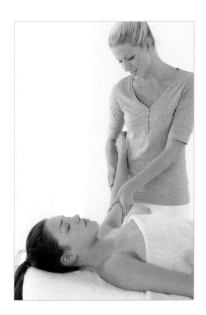

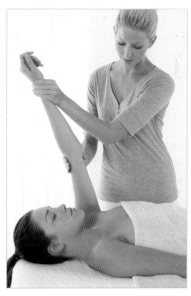

3 squeezing Change the position of your supporting hand to accommodate the squeezing technique over the muscles to the armpit. Pressure should be applied with the web of the hand once more, and should mold to the shape of the arm. Begin the stroke just above the elbow and end just below the armpit, where you should reduce the pressure to avoid sensitivity.

4 pulling After completing the above techniques, lower the arm so that you can adjust your grip. With one hand at the wrist and the other at the elbow, lift the arm to stretch it above your partner's head. Support it just above the elbow joint and stretch the arm up until you feel resistance. Lower the arm, at the same time protecting the elbow, and lie it flat.

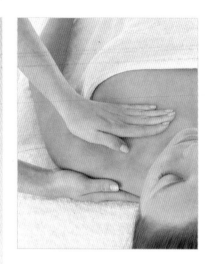

5 squeezing This is a variation of the squeezing technique, using whole-hand contact. Place one hand as far as possible under your partner's shoulder blade and the other on the chest, just below the collarbone. Now apply pressure with both hands and squeeze out toward the arm. This releases the shoulder blade and enables it to lie flatter on the massage surface.

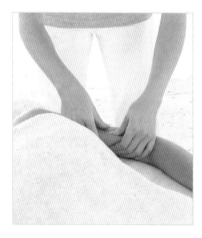

6 kneading This stroke can be a little tricky and you will need to contain your movements. With the arm lying flat, lean across and knead with your fingers over the upper arm muscles. Your movements should be simply over the muscles, and contact should be mostly with the fingers and thumbs. Repeat up and down over the area several times.

7 **thumb pressure** Supporting the elbow from underneath with your fingers, place your thumbs together lengthways and draw them outward over the elbow crease. Reduce your pressure as you complete the stroke. Though simple, this feels wonderfully relaxing and means that the elbow joint does not get left out.

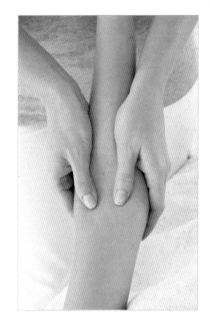

8 **wringing** Lower the arm and place your hands around the forearm, just below the elbow. Now wring with both hands down the arm to the wrist. Keep your hands molded to the shape of the arm, and apply more oil if necessary, so that the stroke feels comfortable over the surface of the skin. Repeat several times.

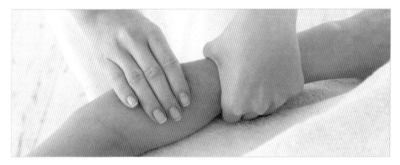

9 thumb pressure Supporting your partner's hand from underneath with your fingers, place your thumbs together over the back of the hand. Draw both thumbs outward over the hand, applying pressure and then releasing it as your thumbs curl toward the palm to complete the stroke. Apply in three different overlapping positions to relax the hand.

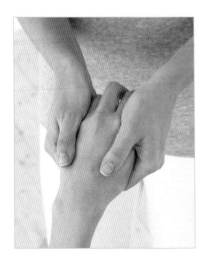

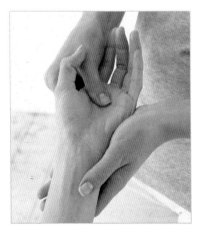

10 thumb-circling Supporting the hand from underneath, press into the palm with the balls of your thumbs, making small circles on the spot. Cover the entire palm, including the base of the fingers and the fleshy area around the thumb. The hands get quite tense, so you can spend some time on these movements, although care is needed around any painful joints.

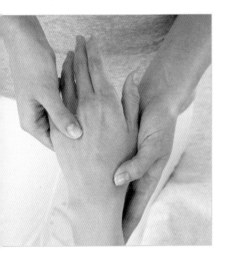

11 squeezing Turning the hand again, place your thumbs and index fingers as high as you can reach on either side of the hand. Draw them slowly down between the tendons and bones until you reach the fingers. Work steadily over the hand until you have completed the movement in each of the four positions. As long as you slide comfortably over the skin, the pressure can be reasonably firm.

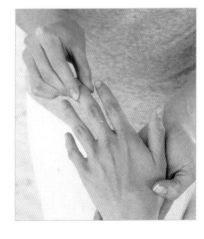

12 pulling Now place your thumb and fingers at the base of your partner's hand and pull each finger in turn. Work thoroughly over the joints and give the tip of each finger a squeeze before completing the movement. Light feathering or rocking is also an option before repeating the sequence on the other arm.

# The chest

Massage on the chest can use broad strokes for a man, but needs to be adapted for a female partner. For men, use additional oil where there is body hair. For women, have a small towel ready to cover the breasts, and always avoid working over the delicate breast tissue.

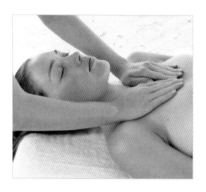

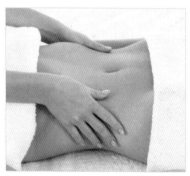

1 **effleurage** Position yourself at your partner's head. Rub some oil between your fingers. Place both hands together flat at the top of your partner's chest. Sweep down the center of the chest to the bottom of the ribcage, avoiding any contact with the breasts. In order to preserve modesty, you can adapt the strokes and use a small towel over the chest instead.

2 **effleurage** Separate your hands at the base of the ribcage, then sweep back up the sides of the body to the armpits. Keep your hands molded to the ribs, at the same time reducing your pressure. Repeat the effleurage strokes several times so that they form one continuous flowing movement.

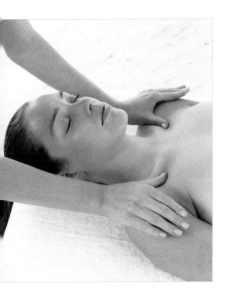

3 thumb pressure Place the balls of both thumbs beneath the collarbone at either side of the sternum (breastbone). Press down and follow the line of the ribs out toward the shoulder. Repeat below the next rib, without applying pressure over the bones. This helps to relax the muscles between the ribs.

4 thumb pressure When working over the chest, it is important to avoid the nipples and breasts. Therefore, in the middle of the chest, you can adapt the strokes by simple thumb pressure between the ribs. Press down with the balls of both thumbs simultaneously, then release the pressure evenly and slowly. Repeat in three to four positions down the center of the ribcage.

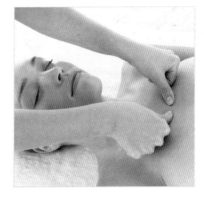

5 finger pressure Place your hands over your partner's ribcage, with the heels on either side of the sternum. Glide out over the ribs using your heels and palms, following the line of the ribs. Then pull back up the sides of the ribcage, with splayed fingers pressing between the bones. Repeat several times in one continuous movement to relax the chest.

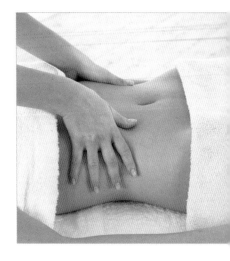

6 heel pressure As you return to the top of the chest, place the heels of your hands on either side of the sternum, just beneath the collarbone. Applying pressure with your heels, draw your hands out toward the shoulders. Repeat under the collarbone several times, easing your pressure as you complete each stroke.

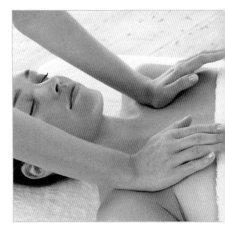

7 finger pressure Reach down to the lower ribs on one side of the body. Place your fingers between the ribs and pull them back over the ribcage, one hand after the other. Sweep both hands up the center of the chest and end the stroke by lightly feathering diagonally over the opposite shoulder. From the same position, repeat on the other side.

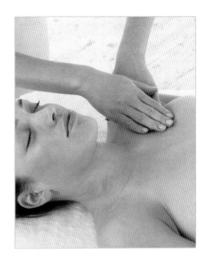

8 heel pressure To end the sequence, place both hands over the tops of the shoulders. Press away from you with the heels of your hands so that your partner's shoulders visibly relax. Repeat, then keep your hands still for a moment, and close the sequence by stroking over the shoulders.

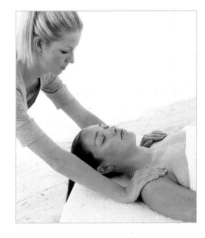

# The abdomen

Massage over the abdomen is very important because it benefits the internal organs as well as helping the body to relax. This area can be emotionally charged and sensitive, so adapt the strokes to your partner's needs and be extra gentle during menstruation. Avoid during pregnancy.

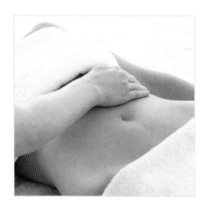

1 effleurage Position yourself at a slight diagonal to your partner. Rub some oil between your fingers, warming it before the first stroke. Place your hands flat over the abdomen and circle around the navel in a clockwise direction. The pressure should be fairly light as this area can be particularly sensitive—the main aim is to spread the oil.

2 circling Now a little more pressure is applied to relax the abdomen. One hand should follow the other so that you circle in a series of flowing movements. Work in a clockwise direction around the navel. Keep whole-hand contact with a relaxed, even pressure to make it feel safe and reassuring. Strokes remain slow.

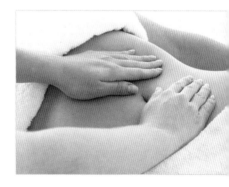

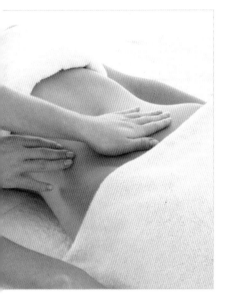

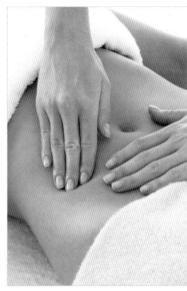

3 circling Follow the circling round until you reach the point where your hands cross. Lift your first hand, cross it over the other, then place it down just in front to continue the strokes. Your second hand should remain in contact. In that way your circling is continuous and the strokes will feel smooth and even.

4 circling Continue the wide, slow circles with one hand to keep the abdomen relaxed, then introduce smaller fingertip circles with the other. The circles should slide over the skin without digging in, and the second hand should follow the first, maintaining the long, slow, relaxing strokes. Work all the way round the navel once.

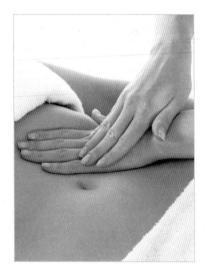
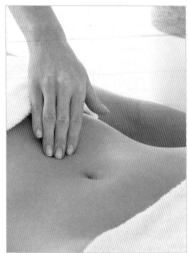

5 palm pressure This movement can be incorporated into your circling strokes. As your hands reach your partner's ribcage, place one hand flat on one side of the body just below the ribs. Press down slowly and evenly, then release your pressure. Continue the circle to the other side of the body, then repeat below the ribs. Be very sensitive to your partner's level of comfort, too little pressure is better than too much.

6 circling Using only your fingers, circle lightly over the solar plexus (the pit of the stomach). This area can get very tense, but is also highly sensitive. Circle in a clockwise direction with flat fingers, with the fingers of your other hand on top to guide the movements if necessary. Concentrate on creating a feeling of relaxation, with warmth radiating out from your hands.

7 wringing Place your hands over your partner's hips, one on either side of the body. Slowly draw your hands toward each other over the abdomen, to reach the opposite side. The main focus is sliding and molding your hands to the hips, with little pressure over the abdomen. Apply more oil if necessary.

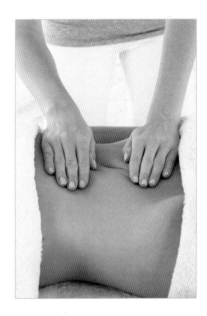

8 energy-sensing To finish the sequence, rest both hands flat over the abdomen, on either side of the navel. Breathe calmly and focus your attention first on your hands, then on your partner's breathing, which should have become deeper and more relaxed. Keep your hands still for a few moments. This will feel comforting and relaxing.

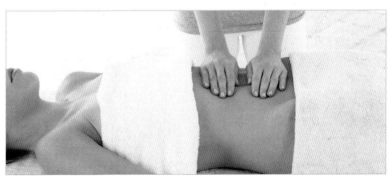

# Front of the legs and feet

This offers the chance to complete your massage by relaxing the muscles, providing a stretch and working right down to the feet. Complete the sequence on each side of the body in turn, using similar pressure. Ending at the feet helps to center the massage.

1 effleurage Position yourself at your partner's foot. Spread some oil over your hands and sweep up the front of the leg, hands together, to the thigh. As you reach the hip, your hands should separate and return down the sides of the leg, with the fingers spread and the pressure reduced. Return to the position just above the ankle and repeat several times.

2 squeezing Place both hands one behind the other, just above the ankle. Gripping with your thumbs and index fingers, squeeze up over the leg toward the knee. Apply pressure to the muscles with the webs between the fingers and thumbs, relaxing your palms so that you reduce the pressure directly over the bone. Stop just below the knee and repeat.

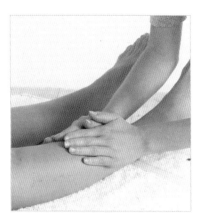

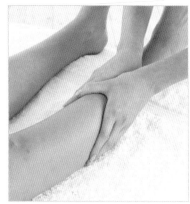

3 squeezing Carry on the squeezing movement up over the thigh, beginning just above the knee. Lean in with your body weight to increase the pressure. Work over the thigh toward the hip several times, avoiding the inner thigh. Spread your thumbs and fingers as wide as you can to accommodate the muscles and increase the effectiveness of the technique.

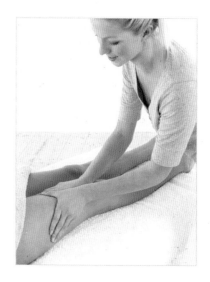

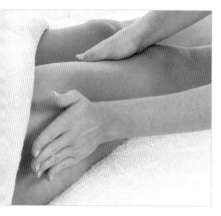

4 heel pressure Change your contact to the heels of your hands to give more pressure over the muscles. One hand should follow the other. As you reach the hip, you can work around the joint using the heel of one hand. Work in circular movements on the spot, applying pressure in toward the hip.

5 kneading Position yourself square on to your partner. Begin kneading movements over the thigh muscles, but avoid the inner thigh. Press into the muscles with your thumbs, pushing slightly away from you, then bring your fingers back toward your thumbs in alternate rhythmic, rolling movements. Work up and down the thigh, ending your strokes above the knee.

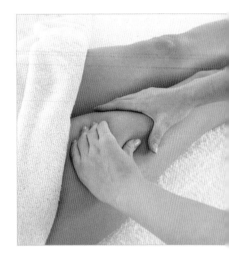

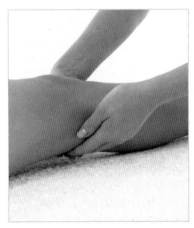

6 rocking Slide your fingers under the knee, and cup the back of the knee with both hands. With the leg slightly bent, rock the joint from side to side while still supporting it with your hands. The leg should be relaxed enough for you to rock without your partner controlling the movement.

7 **wringing** Wring down the leg to the ankle, beginning your movements below the knee. Keep your hands relaxed and molded to the shape of the leg. The wringing movement will feel best when the hands cross right next to each other. Apply more oil as necessary to prevent pulling the skin.

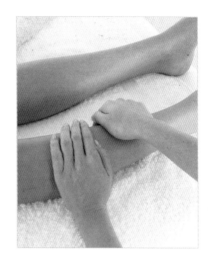

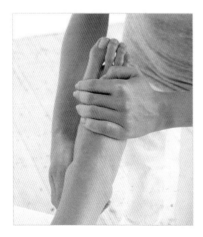

8 **pulling** Place both hands around the ankle, with one hand over the top and the other underneath, cupped around the heel. Lift the leg slightly, then pull back gently toward you to give a good stretch. Only go as far as you can without resistance. Lower the leg carefully afterward.

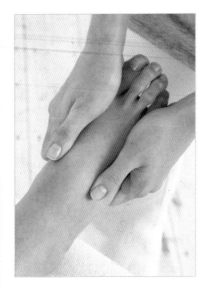

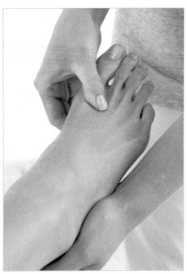

9 thumb pressure Cup your partner's foot in your hand, with your fingers underneath and your thumbs on top. Place the thumbs side by side lengthways in the center of the foot, then slowly draw them apart, sliding outward over the foot. Press with your fingers underneath at the same time so that the foot is slightly arched. Repeat just above the toes.

10 squeezing Reach as far up between the toes as you can, pressing with your thumb and middle finger. Squeeze gently as you draw your hand toward you, until you come to the base of the toes. Repeat in each of the four positions to relax the foot. Use the balls of your finger and thumb to avoid pinching or tickling.

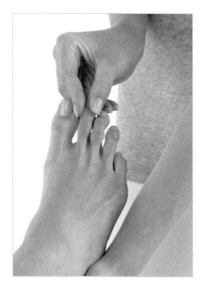

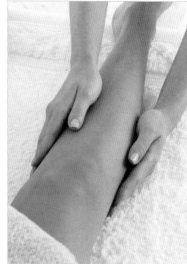

11 squeezing Carry on the squeezing movements with your finger and thumb over each toe in turn. You can rotate the toes and wring the skin slightly with one hand. The other hand supports the foot, cupping around the heel. Continue the movement about 1 in. (2.5 cm) beyond the toes, and finally place the foot down carefully.

12 rocking Moving to the thigh, place your hands on either side of it. Rock with one hand in toward the body, then rock the other way with the other hand. Rock all the way down to the foot and the whole body should respond. Cup your hands over the toes to complete the sequence, then repeat all the movements on the other leg.

# Holistic quick fix

If you only have a few moments for massage, here are four effective steps to help relax the body. Each one should be given as much care and attention as in a whole-body massage for a fully therapeutic experience. Keep to the basic principles and a few careful movements can work wonders.

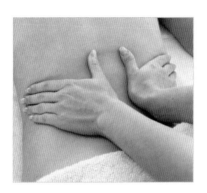

1 thumb pressure on the back
Effleurage over your partner's back to spread the oil. Then press with the balls of your thumbs over the muscles on either side of the spine, going from the upper back all the way down to the lower back. Your pressure and pace should be even from start to finish, with your fingers providing support. Remember not to press over the spine.

2 circling the sacrum Place one hand over the other on the sacrum (the triangle of bone at the base of the spine) and begin slow, counterclockwise circles. Your hands should move evenly over the skin and remain molded to the lower back. Focus on the relaxation process, then rest your hands, with one over your partner's lower back and the other between the shoulder blades.

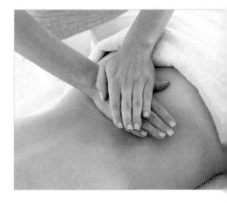

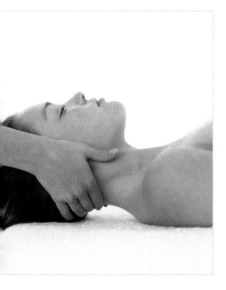

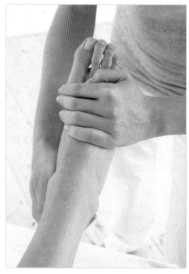

3 **pulling the neck** Ask your partner to turn over. Slide your hands under the neck, then cup both hands at the base of the skull, raise the head slightly, and carefully pull it back toward you. Stop when you feel your partner's resistance. Lower the head and rest your hands for a few moments over your partner's eyes.

4 **pulling the feet** Move to the feet. Grasp one foot with both hands: one over the top and the other supporting it underneath at the heel. Raise the leg slightly, then pull back toward you. Watch the movement in the lower back and hips. When you feel resistance, relax the stretch and lower the leg again. Repeat on the other leg.

# Self-massage

With a little ingenuity, you can apply self-massage to almost any part of your body and experience the benefits that you usually offer to other people. Self-massage also gives you the chance to find points that it may be difficult to locate on a partner without experience.

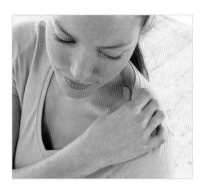 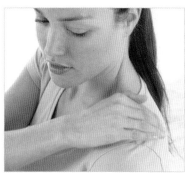

1 **kneading the shoulders** Sitting upright, place one hand over the opposite shoulder and locate the muscle crest along the top. Knead with one hand from the neck out toward the arm and back again. Simply massage the muscles, rather than working over the bone. Press in with your thumb and knead with your fingers until the area feels relaxed. Repeat on the other shoulder.

2 **cupping the shoulders** This is a good way of livening up the muscles. Place one hand over the opposite shoulder, with the palm directly above the muscles. Now cup backward and forward from the neck to the arm, to make the distinctive cupping sound. Keep your hand relaxed with the palm raised, making contact with the heel of your hand and your fingers. The movements should be fairly fast. Repeat on the other shoulder.

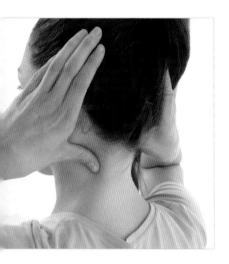

3 thumb pressure on the neck

Place your hands behind your neck, with your thumbs on the muscles on either side of the spine. Make small circles on the spot over the muscles, using your fingertips to provide support. Work slowly up the neck without using too much pressure, until you reach the base of the skull. You should feel your neck relax. If not, repeat the movements.

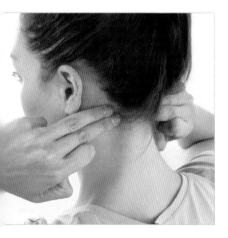

4 finger pressure on the skull

Place both hands at the base of your skull to either side of the spine. Press in under the skull with your middle and fourth fingers, with the hands moving out toward the ears simultaneously. Press in slowly and release equally steadily, using a pressure that feels right. Press at equal distances and stop just behind the ears.

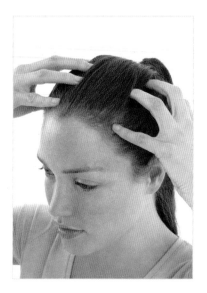

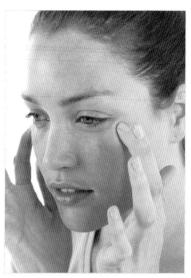

5 rotating over the scalp Place
the fingertips of both hands over your
scalp, then press down and rotate on
the spot with your fingers and thumbs,
using the thumbs as anchors to keep
the fingers steady. Try and get as much
movement as possible. Work right over
the scalp to release any tension, not
forgetting the back of the head and
around the ears.

6 finger pressure on the eye
sockets Use the balls of your middle
fingers to press along the lower eye-
socket ridge. Begin at the bridge of
the nose and work out toward the
temples. Use as much pressure as feels
good to relieve any tension around the
eyes. Press steadily at even distances,
keeping the movements light and fairly
quick. Avoid pulling the skin.

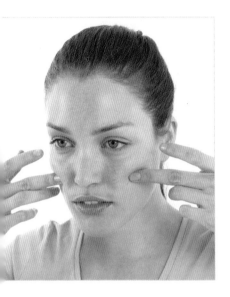

7 **finger pressure under the cheekbones** Use the balls of your middle fingers to press outward under the cheekbones. Begin just beside the nostrils and press in as close to the bone as you can. The movement should be at a slight diagonal upward, under the cheekbones. Press at even distances out toward the jaw. Where the muscles feel tight, circle on the spot to relax them.

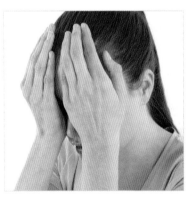

8 **resting the eyes** Place your cupped hands over the eyes to actively rest them. The heels should rest over the cheekbones, the palms should be raised and the fingers should rest on the forehead. This is a great relaxation technique as well as an energy boost. No pressure should be exerted over the eyes, which should be closed for the best results.

9 squeezing the arms It is perfectly possible to perform this technique on yourself. Place your hand just above the elbow of the opposite arm, with the fingers on one side and the thumb on the other. Now squeeze up over the muscles toward the armpit, applying pressure with the web between the index finger and thumb. Repeat several times, then repeat on the opposite arm.

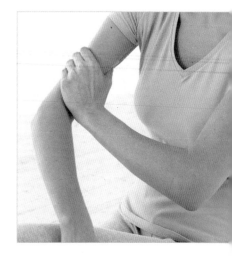

10 pummelling the hips Form your hands into loose fists and use them to pummel over your buttocks and hips. This is an invigorating movement designed to stimulate circulation in an area where the muscles and joints can get quite tight. Use as much pressure as you need, keeping the movements lively. Use your hands alternately to establish a good rhythm.

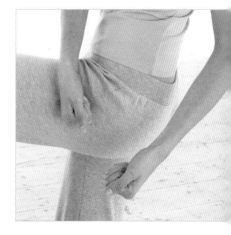

11 **squeezing the legs** For this movement you need to be flexible enough to reach your calf. Bend your leg and cup your hands around the calf muscles, with the fingers at the front and the thumbs behind. Now use your thumbs to squeeze up over the calf toward the knee, where no pressure should be applied. Your fingers should act as a support to steady the movement. Repeat on the other leg.

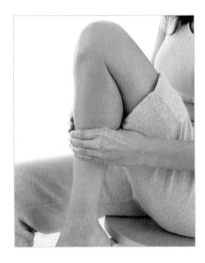

12 **thumb pressure on the feet**
Here you need to be flexible enough to reach the sole of your foot. Bend your leg and place the balls of your thumbs on the sole of your foot, with the fingers supporting it over the top. Work over the sole using small circular movements, with your thumbs working alternately. Avoid the instep and concentrate on the ball of the foot and base of the toes. Repeat on the other foot.

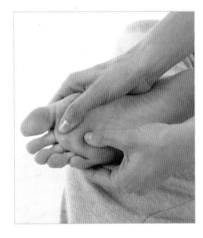

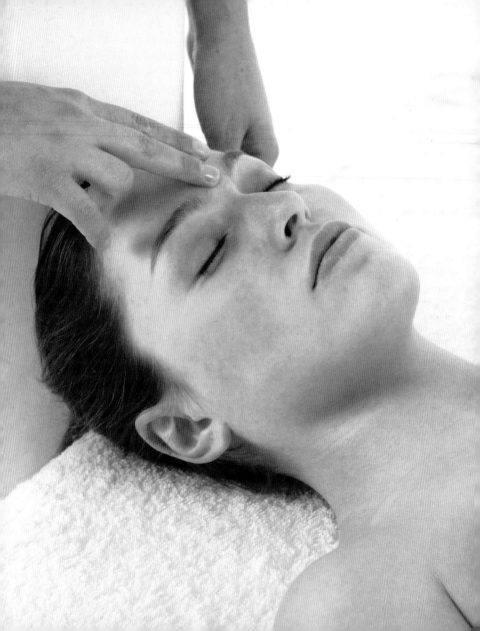

# Chinese massage

Chinese massage is a combination of techniques
to improve the flow of energy (*chi*) within the
body and increase vitality. In this Chinese massage
sequence, strokes to relax the muscles and stimulate
the meridians (energy channels) combine with
acupressure over the points. The aim is to balance
and energize your partner. The quality of your touch
and movements is more important than exact point
location, which takes time, requires feedback, and
becomes easier with practice and experience. So
work with an open mind.

# Principles

Chinese massage, or *TuiNa*, is based on an oriental approach to the body and health. It is a comprehensive, holistic approach, which takes into account not only the individual, but also interaction between the individual and the environment. All elements are important in diagnosis.

Traditional Chinese medicine includes a number of complex systems, and the relationships between its various elements are of great importance.

## The meridians

According to Chinese principles, there are various channels of energy, or meridians, throughout the body. They number 12 pairs on either side of two central channels, making a total of 14 meridians. In addition, there are a further six extraordinary meridians. All these channels circulate *chi* (internal vital energy), and good health depends on a harmonious balance of *chi* between the different meridians.

Harmony not only needs to exist within the body, but also in the interchange between the individual and the external world. Exchanges of energy are constantly taking place, and once again balance is the key. According to traditional Chinese philosophy, the world is composed of the interplay between opposites, known as *yin* and *yang* (see also page 202); and an imbalance of *yin* and *yang* within the body can be seen as either an excess or deficiency of *chi*.

Each of the meridians is governed by a particular body organ and has particular characteristics. The two central meridians, which are of special importance, are known as the Conception Vessel (CV, which runs up the front of the body and is predominantly *yin* in character) and the Governor Vessel (GV, which runs up the back and is predominantly *yang*).

*This 18th-century Chinese illustration shows the position of the points along the Governor Vessel channel.*

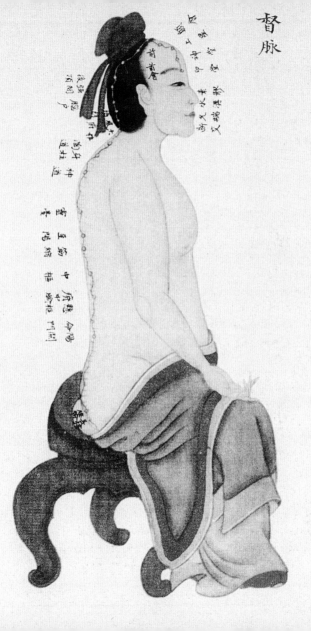

# Acupressure points

An almost bewildering number of acupressure points are located within the body. Each lies on a particular meridian, but the 14 meridians are of varying lengths and so have different numbers of points. Each point is known by the meridian on which it is located and by its number in the sequence.

While some meridians (such as the gallbladder meridian) begin in the upper body, others begin in the extremities and work upward. For example, KI—the first point along the kidney meridian—is located in the foot. The bladder meridian is the longest, with 67 points along its length.

*Chi* flows from one meridian to another, as well as between the points. Stimulation of the points may be done by needles (as in acupuncture) or by fingers and thumbs (as in *TuiNa*). While pressure via the hands may be less accurate, the principles remain the same. The aim is to relieve blockages of energy within the channels and to assist the flow of *chi*. This in turn will affect the functioning of the organs and will help return the body to health.

A full assessment normally precedes massage, including oriental pulse and tongue diagnosis. While it takes the training of a skilled practitioner to address medical problems, Chinese massage is a great way to aid relaxation and maintain good health. Knowledge of a few principal points (see pages 161–163) is a good way to begin, and location of the points is achieved by measuring in finger-widths relative to the person you are massaging, or with the thumb. Each thumb measurement is known as one *cun*.

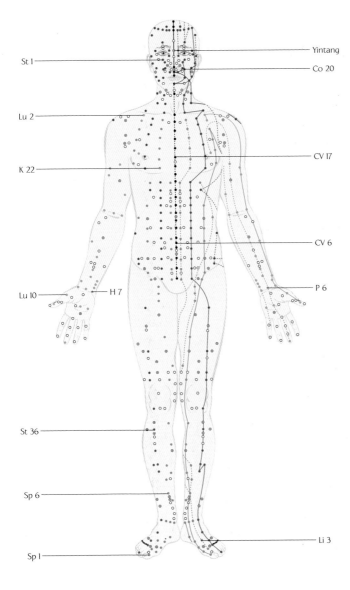

Yintang

St 1

Co 20

Lu 2

CV 17

K 22

CV 6

Lu 10 — H 7

P 6

St 36

Sp 6

Li 3

Sp 1

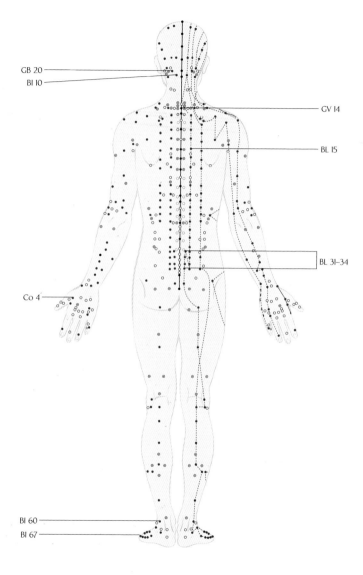

GB 20

Bl 10

GV 14

BL 15

BL 31–34

Co 4

Bl 60

Bl 67

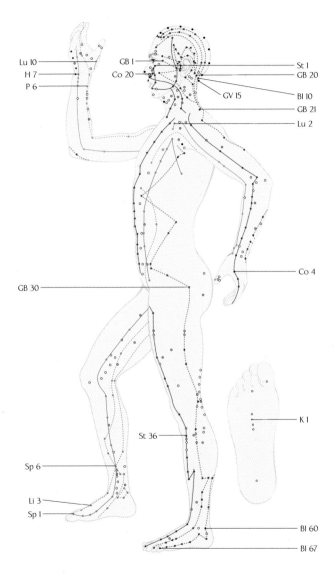

Lu 10
H 7
P 6
GB 1
Co 20
St 1
GB 20
GV 15
Bl 10
GB 21
Lu 2
Co 4
GB 30
K 1
St 36
Sp 6
Li 3
Sp 1
Bl 60
Bl 67

# Application

Chinese medicine refers to two types of *chi* within the body: the *chi* you are born with (known as "before-heaven *chi*"), which is stored in the kidneys and may be weak or become depleted in some people and is difficult to restore; and "after-heaven *chi*," which flows throughout the body.

*Chi* can be influenced by, for example, diet, fresh air, or lifestyle; it should flow freely through the meridians, nourishing and supporting the body. Blockage of this flow can result in an excess, deficiency, or stagnation of *chi*, whose effects may be felt as pain, swelling, or inflammation. Stimulating the flow of energy and dispersing the build-up of *chi* helps to increase vitality and return the body to balance and good health.

Traditionally, Chinese massage was performed clothed, through a sheet to

## FOCUS POINTS

**Techniques:** The main techniques are effleurage, elbow pressure, thumb-rolling, thumb and finger pressure, stretching, and rocking.

**Movements:** These vary between flowing, stimulating, and pressure movements, and should follow on from each other to give the massage shape and form.

**Equipment:** You need a firm surface, such as a massage table or soft mat on the floor; towels to cover the area you are not working on; supports for the head, knees, or ankles; and some oil (see pages 30–33).

**Feedback:** Make a note of any problems before starting, and ask your partner for feedback about the location and especially any tenderness associated with the acupressure points.

**Timing:** A whole-body *TuiNa* massage should take about 45 minutes.

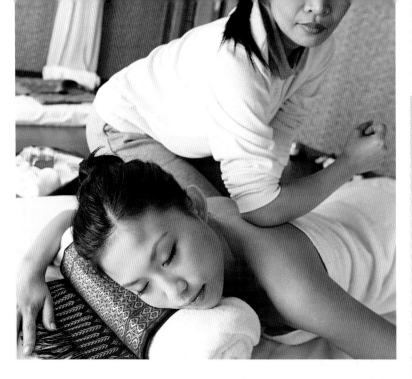

preserve the recipient's modesty. However, oil can be used so that the strokes relax the muscles as well as working along the meridians. Pressure to stimulate the points is done mainly with the thumbs and fingers. For deeper movements the balls of the thumbs and elbows may be used, and for lighter, vibrating stimulation the fingertips are excellent. Care should be taken to listen to the body and use pressure that is appropriate. Movements may need to

*In Chinese massage, thumbs, fingers, and elbows are used to stimulate energy flow and promote the flow of chi.*

be either quick and light or deeper and slower. When giving a massage, try to stay in tune with your own body and this will be conveyed to your partner. Being correctly positioned (see pages 34–35) will enable you to focus on sensitivity. Massage around, rather than over, painful areas to disperse energy.

# The back

Position yourself so that you can reach the back comfortably, with everything you need to hand. Center yourself first, then begin massage on the back, which will have an effect on the whole body. The techniques include both massage and the use of pressure points.

1 effleurage Spread some oil over your hands. Position yourself at your partner's head and glide your hands together down to the lower back. You can apply relatively firm pressure with your palms. The aim is to wake up the meridians. Spread your fingers at the lower back and draw them back up either side of the ribs to the shoulders. Repeat briskly several times.

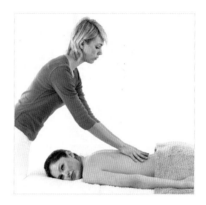

2 circling Move to the side. Place your thumbs on either side of the spine and circle over the muscles by the prominent vertebra (C7) at the base of the neck. This point is known as GV 14 and the circling movements help to relax the neck. As you circle, imagine any tension releasing out toward the shoulders. Repeat slowly several times.

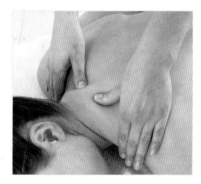

3 squeezing Return to the head.
Place your thumbs over GB 21, which
is located in the depression midway
between C7 and the shoulder. Position
your fingers over your partner's
shoulders and squeeze several times.
This helps to relax the shoulders. If the
point is sore, massage around it with
the thumbs to disperse excess *chi*.

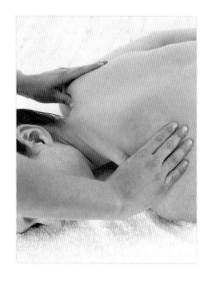

**CAUTION**

Do not use point GB 21
during pregnancy.

4 thumb-rolling Place both your
thumbs on the ridge of muscles to one
side of the spine. Roll with the thumbs,
alternating your strokes down to the
lower back. This relaxes the bladder
meridian, which lies on either side of
the spine. Your strokes can be fairly
brisk. Repeat several times, then repeat
on the other side.

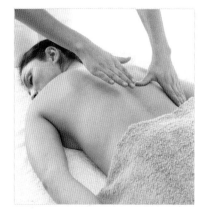

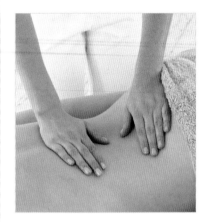

5 palm pressure Move to your partner's lower back and apply a little oil. Place one hand flat over the sacrum (the triangle of bone at the base of the spine) and the other across the lower back. Cup your upper hand slightly so that there is no pressure over the spine. Anchoring with the upper hand, carefully stretch over the muscles with the other palm to relax the lower back. Repeat with sensitivity.

6 palm pressure Repeat the movement, this time over the lower back muscles on either side of the spine. Lean over your partner and cup both hands over the muscles, avoiding any pressure on the spine. Then stretch with one hand toward the shoulders and the other to the hip. This relaxes the powerful muscles along the bladder meridian and helps to ease the lower back. Repeat several times.

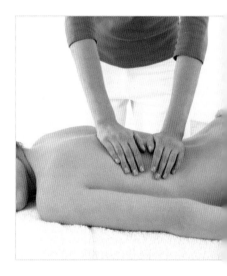

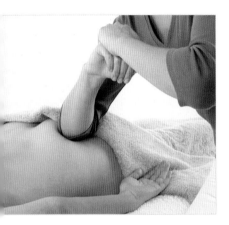

7 **elbow pressure** Move to one of
your partner's hips. Locate GB 30 with
your fingers, one-third of the way
down the buttock and two-thirds
toward the hip. Guide your elbow
to the point with your fingers, then
slowly press in toward the hip, keeping
your elbow rounded. Release and then
repeat. This area can be tight and
extremely sensitive, but stimulation is
good for relaxing the hip. Your partner
should breathe calmly to relax. Repeat
the last two movements on the
other side.

8 **thumb pressure** Return your
hands to the lower back. Place both
thumbs roughly 1½ in. (4 cm) away
from the spine on either side of the
sacrum. Press Bl 31–34 with both
thumbs simultaneously, locating the
little depressions in the bone. Press
each point gently once, then release
and move on to the next point.

**CAUTION**

Do not use points Bl 31–34
during pregnancy.

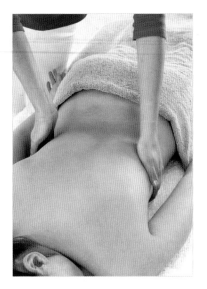

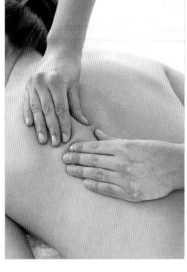

9 rocking Place both hands on either side of your partner's ribs. Gently rock the body away from you, then rock back again the other way with your other hand. Continue with alternate movements down to the hips. Repeat toward the armpits and back one final time to the hips. This helps to relax the entire back.

10 squeezing Position yourself at the shoulders. Place your thumbs at one side of the muscles to the side of the spine, with your fingers in the same position on the other side. Squeeze into the muscles with your fingers and thumbs, and squeeze toward the spine. Move along the muscles from the upper to the lower back, making sure that your fingers do not dig in. Repeat on the opposite side of the spine.

11 thumb pressure Use the balls of
your thumbs to press into the muscles
either side of the spine. Pressing
between the shoulder blades, stimulate
Bl 15. This should be nice and relaxed, so
circle around the points on both sides
until you feel a reduction in muscle tone.
Return to the point once more and press
in evenly again with your thumbs.

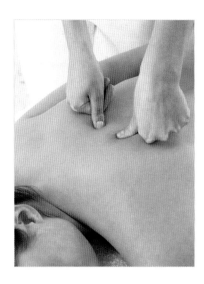

12 firm stroking To finish the back
sequence, place both hands flat against
the sides of your partner's body. Draw
your hands down to the hips. Repeat
twice more, fairly vigorously, to draw
the *yang* energy down the back.

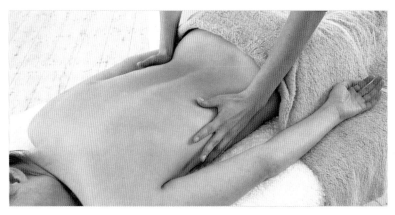

# Back of the legs and feet

This sequence continues massage over the meridians, combined with specific pressure points for the legs and feet. Complete working on one side of the body before beginning the sequence on the other. Your pressure and pace should be similar for each leg.

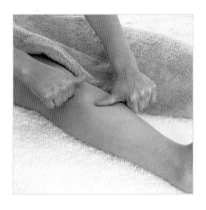

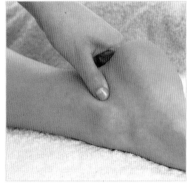

1 thumb-rolling Rub some oil between your hands and effleurage over your partner's leg. This helps the massage movements. Then roll your thumbs from thigh to ankle, following the bladder meridian, which lies along the middle of the thigh and ends just behind the ankle bone. Do not use pressure over the back of the knee. Repeat, alternating the thumb rolls several times.

2 thumb pressure Squeeze Bl 60, which is level with and just behind the ankle joint. Apply pressure with your thumb for a few moments and release.

CAUTION

Do not use point Bl 60 during pregnancy.

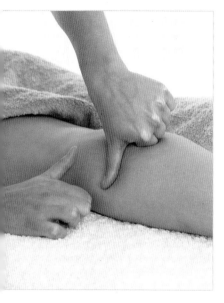

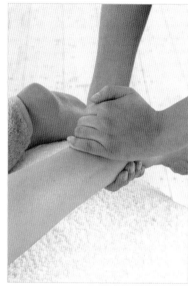

3 **thumb-rolling** Move to the outer thigh and repeat the rolling movements down the leg, again avoiding pressure over the back of the knee. Follow the gall-bladder meridian fairly briskly down to the ankle joint. Massage as if you are rolling energy down the leg. Repeat the movements several times.

4 **pulling** Move to the foot and grasp your partner's leg, with one hand underneath and the other above the heel. Lift the leg carefully and pull it gently toward you. Rock the leg slightly as you put it down, to stimulate the flow of energy.

5 thumb-circling Support your partner's feet with both hands and place your thumbs over KI in the middle, just under the ball of the foot. This is good for boosting energy. Circle on the spot with both thumbs simultaneously, increasing the pressure as you do so. Circling rather than pressing spreads the pressure over a wider area.

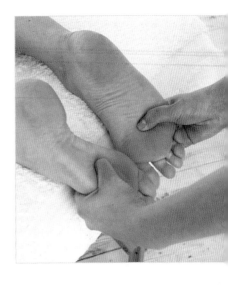

### CAUTION

Do not use points KI or BI 67 during pregnancy.

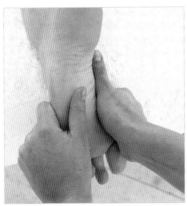

6 squeezing Pick up your partner's foot and place your hands on either side. Squeeze it between the fingers and thumbs. Now squeeze one side of the foot toward you, while squeezing the other side away. This helps to release tension in the foot. Squeeze up and down until the muscles feel looser.

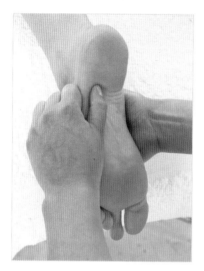

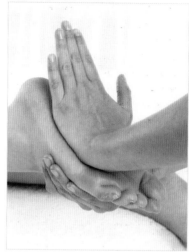

7 squeezing Support the foot with your hand, squeezing along the outside with the thumb and fingers. Use fairly firm pressure. Squeeze and pinch from the heel along the fleshy part of the foot to the little toe. Repeat several times, then squeeze Bl 67 at the corner of the little toe nailbed and pull your fingers away quickly with a little snap.

8 rubbing Pick up the foot and rub the ball of it between your hands. Pay particularly attention to the KI point, which you massaged before (see Step 5). You can rub quite vigorously. Place the foot down, then pull the toes one by one to release the *chi* and repeat the whole sequence on the other leg.

# Front of the legs and feet

The massage sequence continues upward from the feet and legs, following the direction of the meridians. The work is on the acupressure channels and points, some of which are stimulated specifically. Massage each side of the body in turn, keeping the pressure similar and consistent.

1 **thumb-rolling** Rub some oil over your hands. Roll up the inside of your partner's leg with your thumbs, beginning your movements just above the ankle. Apply reasonably firm pressure at a fairly vigorous pace. Carefully work around the fleshy inner side of the knee, then stop just above. Repeat several times, but check the comfort levels with your partner because these points can be sensitive.

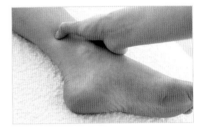

2 **thumb pressure** Return to the ankle and locate Spl 6, three finger-widths up from the ankle joint, just behind the bone. Proceed cautiously as this point can be extremely tender, especially for women. Press gently and, if the point is sore, circle on the spot to disperse the *chi*.

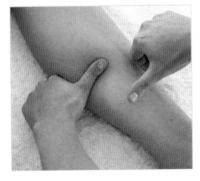

### CAUTION

Do not use point Spl 6 during pregnancy.

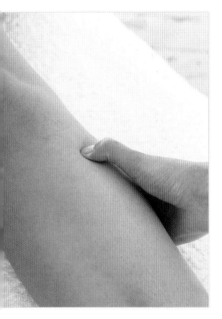
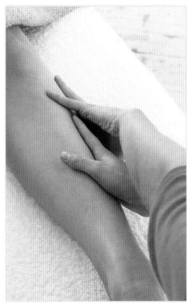

3 **thumb pressure** Cross to the other side of the leg and find St 36, which lies at the outer edge of the shinbone, three finger-widths below the knee. Press with your thumb, starting gently and then increasing the pressure. Hold for a few moments and then release. This is a good digestive tonic.

4 **stroking** Stroke down the length of the outer leg at the end of this sequence to bring the *chi* to the feet. Use the flats of your hands and fingertips fairly briskly, stroking down to the ankle joint. Repeat the movements several times, then position yourself at your partner's feet.

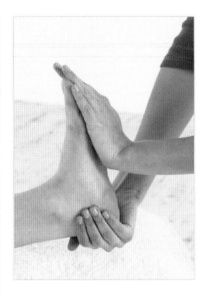

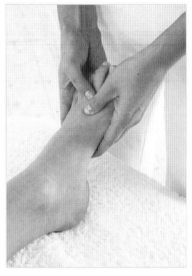

5  rotating Grasp the sole of your partner's foot with one hand while supporting underneath the leg with the other. Rotate the ankle joint several times in both directions, then press the entire foot directly back toward the body as far as your partner's flexibility will allow. This helps to release stiffness in the ankle.

6  thumb-rolling Support the foot from underneath and locate Li 3, which lies in the depression between the big and first toes. Roll your thumbs in small alternating movements over the point, stroking up toward the ankle. Repeat several times. This should feel quite relaxing, and is a good tonic point.

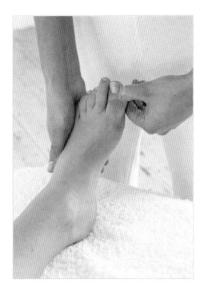

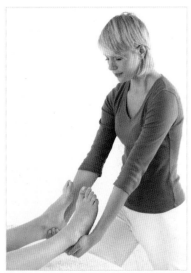

7 **thumb pressure** Move to the
big toe. Holding it with one hand to
provide resistance, press at the outer
corner of the nail with the side of your
thumb. This stimulates Sp 1, which is
good for nourishing energy. Press into
the point and release. Then repeat all
the movements on the other leg.

8 **rocking** Stand at the feet and slide
your hands under both of your
partner's ankles. Lift the legs slightly
and gently rock, pulling toward you as
you do so. Keep your shoulders relaxed.
This aligns the body and helps the flow
of energy. Place the legs back down
and pause for a moment before
breaking contact with your partner.

# The arms and hands

Position yourself so that you can comfortably massage the length of the arms. Bear in mind the directions of the meridians at both the front and back of the arms. Work on the hands and fingers is important in helping to release excess *chi*.

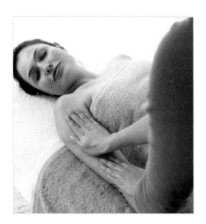

1 effleurage Rub some oil over your hands and effleurage down the inside of your partner's arm, following the lung meridian from the chest downward over the ball of the shoulder. Stroke down the arm several times, returning up the back of the arm. Repeat using greater pressure on the downward stroke.

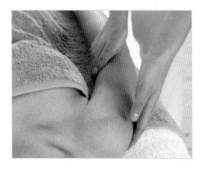

2 rocking Cup your hands under the shoulder and, supporting the arm, rock gently down the arm to the hand. Both hands should remain in contact for the length of the stroke. This helps to relax the arm muscles and shoulder joint. Repeat the movement several times, then squeeze firmly down to the hand.

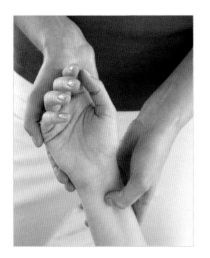

3 thumb pressure Support the arm with one hand. P6 is located between the tendons, two and a half finger-widths above the wrist. Place your thumb over the point, pressing gently with the ball, and continue the pressure until your partner feels the connection. Hold for a few moments and then release slowly. This is good for regulating the circulation.

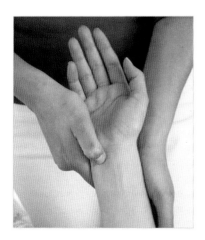

4 thumb pressure Move your thumb to the little-finger side of the wrist. In a line down from the inside of the little finger you will find a depression just by the bone, which is H7. Place your thumb over the point and press carefully with the tip, close in to the bone. Continue with the pressure until you connect with the point, then release the pressure evenly.

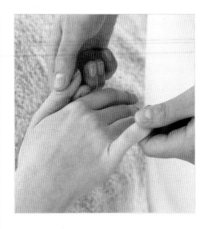

5 rocking Hold your partner's hand by the little finger and thumb, then lift the forearm slightly and rock gently from side to side, to relax both the wrist and finger joints. Lower the arm, let your partner relax, then try again. This time the hand should feel much looser.

6 thumb pressure Place your thumb over the web of your partner's hand between the thumb and index finger, supporting it from underneath. Locate the soft depression and press in gently to Co 4 with the tip of your thumb. Increase the pressure slowly because this can be a sensitive point. It is good for the digestion and headaches.

CAUTION

Do not use point Co 4 during pregnancy.

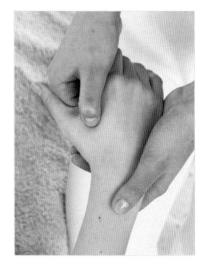

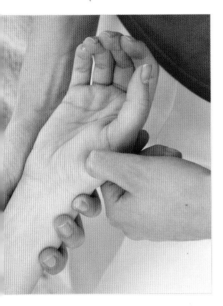

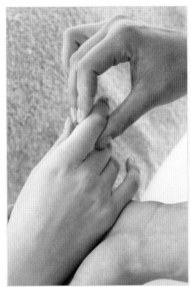

7 **thumb pressure** Turn the hand over and locate Lu 10, which lies halfway down the fleshy part of the thumb. Press with the tip of your thumb diagonally in toward the bone. You can apply reasonable pressure over this point. Hold for a few moments, then release.

8 **squeezing** Supporting the hand, squeeze and twist the length of each finger and the thumb in turn. Use your thumb, index, and middle fingers for a good grip. This relaxes the joints, stimulates the meridians and points in the hand, and releases *chi* from the body. Then repeat all the movements on the other arm.

# The chest

Apply sensitivity when massaging the chest because this area can be quite emotionally charged. For a female partner you may need a towel to cover the breasts, which should not be worked on directly. As a general rule, apply less pressure over vulnerable areas of the body.

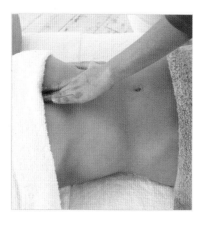

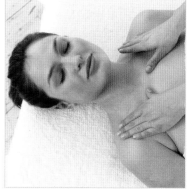

1 finger pressure Roll with your thumbs up to your partner's chest, and locate CV 17, which is on the breastbone, at the midpoint between the nipples. Place your middle finger over the point and press gently, slowly increasing the pressure toward the chest. Hold for a moment, then release. This is good to regulate the emotions, as well as for the general constitution.

2 thumb-rolling Continue by rolling with both thumbs up the center of the chest, working toward the collarbone. Separate your thumbs so that they fan out over the ribs as far as Lu 2, which is located about one finger-width below the collarbone and six finger-widths from the center of the chest. Repeat the fanning movements between the ribs several times.

3 thumb pressure Roll up the center of the abdomen again, this time separating your thumbs under the ribcage. Locate K22, which lies two finger-widths out from the center of the chest, just beneath the breasts. Use both thumbs to circle over the points, then release.

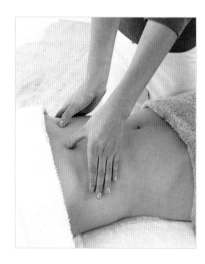

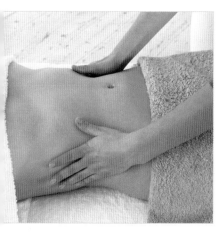

4 stroking Fan your hands out to the sides of the body and lie the palms flat against either side of the ribcage. Draw your hands down to the hips, fingers splayed, applying slight pressure as you do so. Repeat several times to draw *chi* toward the feet.

# The abdomen

Work on the abdomen should soothe and center your partner. Position yourself so that you are relaxed and comfortable before you begin the sequence. Be sensitive during your partner's menstruation, when you might only want to use Step 4. During pregnancy only use Step 4.

1 **effleurage** Rub some oil between your hands and effleurage over your partner's abdomen in a clockwise direction. This spreads the oil, but is also an opportunity to help the abdomen relax. Keep the hands soft and flat and molded to your partner's body. However, if your partner is suffering from diarrhea, circle counterclockwise.

2 **circling** Continue circling with the hands flat against the abdomen, but this time circle over each part several times to fully relax it. The hand circles should be full and generous and the movements continuous. This technique is known as *mofa* and involves lots of circles around the abdomen to activate the large intestine.

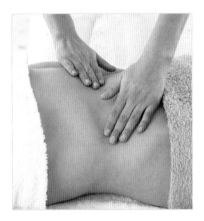

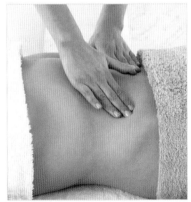

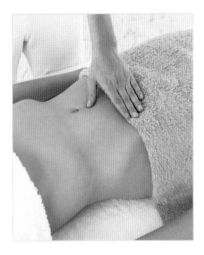

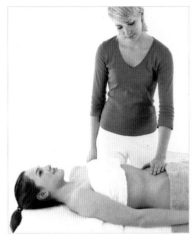

3 thumb pressure Locate CV 6,
which is the point approximately two
finger-widths below the navel, lying in
the central line of the body. Hold your
thumb over the point, then start
pressing it gently. Check that the
pressure feels okay with your partner.
Hold for a moment, then release
steadily and evenly. This should be
done with care on women.

CAUTION

Do not use point CV 6
during pregnancy.

4 resting Rest your hand over the
Tan Den point—this is located roughly
2 in. (5 cm) below the navel and one-
third of the way toward the spine;
in Chinese philosophy it is a very
important energy point for centring
the body. Focus your attention on
the palm of your hand. Breathe calmly
and observe the rise and fall of your
partner's breath. The warmth of your
hand will provide comfort and focus
your partner's attention on this very
important central point.

# The neck and scalp

Work with slow, steady, supportive movements to help your partner relax. Relaxing the neck is very important, but most people find it hard to let go. Repeat the movements over the muscles as necessary until you feel a change in muscle tone.

1 rocking Move to your partner's head. Slide your hands under the neck, cup your hands at the base of the skull and lift the head slightly. Gently rock from side to side to relax the neck. If your partner has difficulty relaxing, lower the head gently, wait for a moment and then try again. Stop if you feel any resistance or there is any pain.

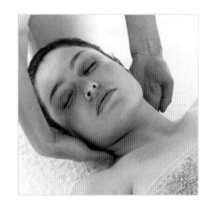

2 finger pressure Cupping the head in your hands, carefully turn it to one side. This movement should be smooth and reassuring. Locate Bl 10, which is in the depression just below the base of the skull, roughly two finger-widths out from the spine. Press with the balls of your index and middle fingers once, then release.

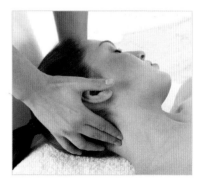

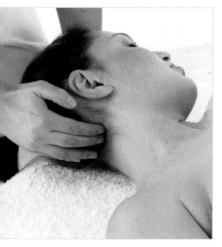

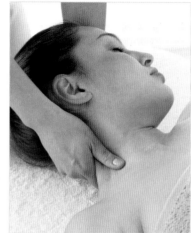

3 finger pressure Turn the head toward the shoulder a little more and locate GB 20, which is a further two finger-widths out from the spine, in the depression at the base of the skull. Press with the balls of your index and middle fingers, keeping the pressure steady and even. This relieves tension around the head and neck.

4 squeezing Still supporting your partner's head with your hand, squeeze along the neck muscles, using your fingers and the heel of your hand. Work from the shoulders up to the base of the skull. You can squeeze reasonably firmly as you work along the top of the shoulder. Then repeat all the movements by turning the head and working on the opposite side.

5 squeezing Squeeze both of your partner's ears between your fingers and thumbs. Follow the shape of the ears, working round the outside to the lobes three times. Repeat the movements a further three times in a second line around the inside of the ears. Your movements should be a series of light simultaneous pinches.

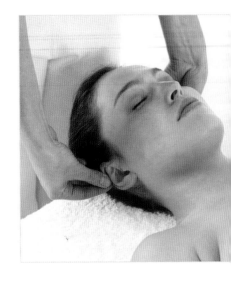

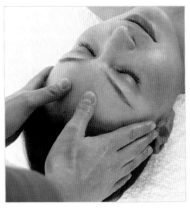

6 thumb pressure Press with both thumbs in a line up from the inner brow to the hairline and continue over the back of the head. The pressure should be quick and light, using the balls of both thumbs at the same time. Take care to hold your fingers away from the face. Repeat several times to clear any congestion.

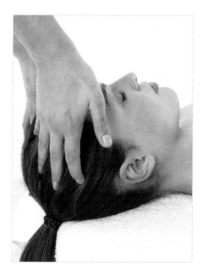

7 **finger pressure** Turn your palms to face the back of your partner's head and rake the balls of your fingers through the hair. Work over the scalp in several lines until you have covered as much of the head as you can reasonably reach.

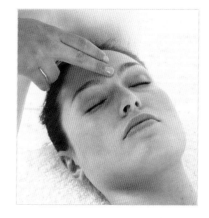

8 **finger pressure** Return to the forehead and locate the Yintang point, which lies between the brows. Hold your middle finger in place, then press lightly to relax and calm the mind. This should be done slowly and sensitively. Hold for a few seconds and breathe calmly yourself, then release it.

# The face

Finishing the sequence on the face makes a calming end to the massage. The pressure can be reasonably firm as the aim is stimulation of the meridians and pressure points; and it can be even firmer on a man's skin. By the end of the massage you should both feel more energized.

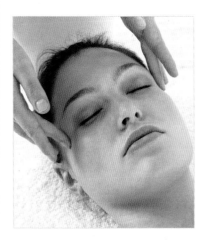

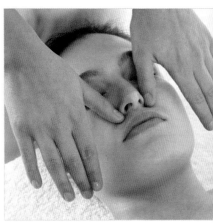

1 finger pressure Place the balls of your fingers over your partner's temples, then locate the small depressions approximately one finger-width away from the eye sockets. Carefully press GB 1 with the tips of your middle fingers. Begin slowly until you feel the energy of each point, hold for a moment and then release.

2 thumb pressure Place your thumbs just below the side of each nostril and locate the depression where Co 20 lies. It should be quite easy to find. Press in a slight diagonal toward the nose, using the sides of your thumbs. This is good for the sinus. Hold for a moment, then release your pressure.

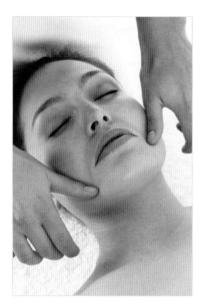
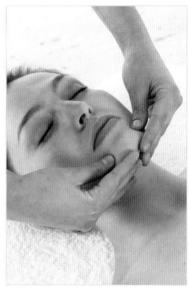

3 thumb-rolling Rub a little oil over your fingers and roll your thumbs in a diagonal line from the nostrils out toward the jaw. The strokes should be made with both thumbs at once on either side of the face. Repeat several times with enough pressure so that you can see your partner's skin move.

4 thumb-rolling Place your thumbs at the outer corners of the lips and roll diagonally with the sides of your thumbs to the jawline. Use both thumbs at once. Repeat several times, and end the strokes by gently cupping your hands under the jaw.

# Chinese massage quick fix

The following are some important points to work on, for a mini Chinese massage that will not take long to complete and that offers good tension release. Focus as you would on a whole body massage. The points selected both relax and provide a tonic to the system.

1 circling the back Rub a little oil between your fingers, and then effleurage in fanning movements over your partner's upper back. Find the prominent vertebra just below the level of the shoulders and circle over the muscles at either side of GV 14, in the central line of the body. Try and release any neck tension out toward the shoulders, then continue effleurage down the back.

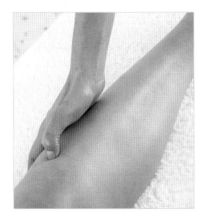

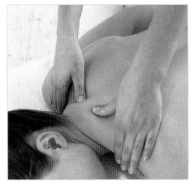

2 thumb pressure on the legs Once your partner has turned over, locate St 36 by running your hand up the shinbone until you feel the depression three finger-widths below the knee. Press gently with the ball of your thumb, and circle on the spot to relax the area, before increasing your pressure. Hold for a few moments, then release.

3 thumb-rolling the feet Cup your
fingers under the foot for support and
locate Li 3 between the big and first
toes. Roll both thumbs over the point
alternately to disperse the *chi*, stroking
in the direction of the ankle. The
movements should be quite gentle and
repetitive, and the thumb rolls should
be small. Repeat a number of times,
then repeat the last two movements
on the other leg.

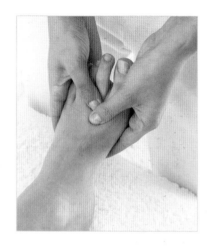

4 thumb pressure on the arms
Locate P6, which is in the center of
the arm between the tendons, two and
a half finger-widths above the wrist.
Supporting the wrist from underneath,
press with the ball of your thumb,
starting gently and increasing the
pressure slowly. Hold for a few
moments, then release and repeat
on the other arm.

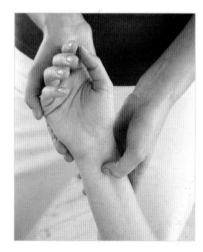

# Self-massage

Self-massage is a great way of locating points that can be difficult to find on other people without a bit of practice. The points may feel a little tender, and you will feel the energy resonate when you have found the right spot. The more you practice, the more natural it becomes.

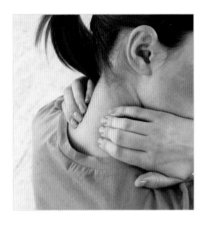

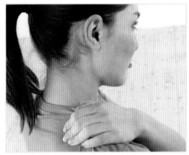

2 squeezing the shoulders Reach over your shoulder and squeeze the muscles between your fingers and the heel of your hand. Squeeze toward the neck, and locate GB 21, which is in a line with GV 14. You will feel a tender depression. Circle on the spot with your fingertips, then press directly a little harder. Repeat the movements on the other shoulder.

1 finger-circling the shoulders The neck and shoulders always get tense, so this is a good way to relax. Reach over your shoulders and locate the muscles on either side of GV 14. Circle with your fingertips as firmly as feels comfortable, in order to relax them. Fan them out across the back toward the arms to disperse any build-up of *chi*.

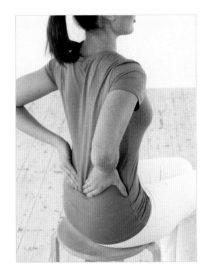

3 **finger pressure on the lower back** Place your hands behind your back, with the fingertips over the lower back muscles on either side of the spine. Push your fingers down the muscles and over the sacrum, the bony triangle at the base of the spine. This stimulates the bladder meridian and is a good way of relaxing the lower back.

### CAUTION

Do not use points GV 14, GB 21, or GB 30 during pregnancy.

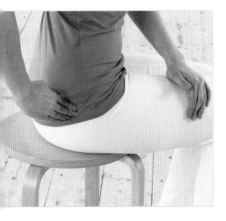

4 **finger pressure on the buttocks** Locate GB 30, which is two-thirds of the way over the buttocks toward the hip and about one-third of the way down. Press in and circle with the tips of your fingers. Although it is hard to achieve the same pressure on yourself as on a partner, you can still relax the hip area quite well.

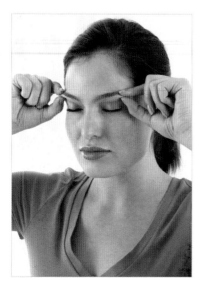

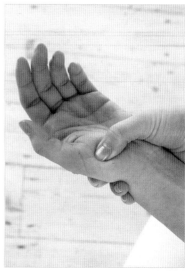

5 **squeezing the eyebrows** Pinch across the line of the eyebrows with your thumbs and index fingers, moving from the bridge of the nose out toward the temples. Pinch and lift as you do so, working your way over to GB 1. You can feel this depression in a line leading out from the eye socket. Pressing and circling here is great for relieving tension and waking up tired eyes.

6 **thumb pressure** Support one hand in the other and massage over the fleshy part of the thumb. Your fingers provide resistance from underneath. Locate Lu 10, which is halfway down the fleshy part of the thumb. Circle and then press in gently with the tip of your active thumb, pressing toward the bone. Hold for a moment, then release and repeat on the other hand.

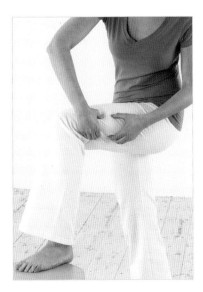

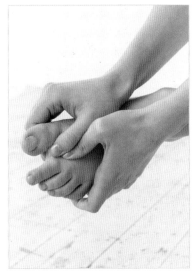

7 **squeezing the legs** Pinch and squeeze down the outside of both legs from the tops of the thighs to the ankles. Apply pressure between your thumbs and fingers, and make your movements brisk and vigorous. Avoid any pressure over the knees. Repeat several times to draw the energy to the ground.

8 **thumb pressure on the toes** Supporting the foot from underneath, place one thumb over the opposite foot in the web between the first and big toes. Locate Li 3 and press it with the tip of your thumb. This point can be quite sensitive, so you can circle on the spot to disperse the pressure, then try pressing it directly again. Repeat on the other side.

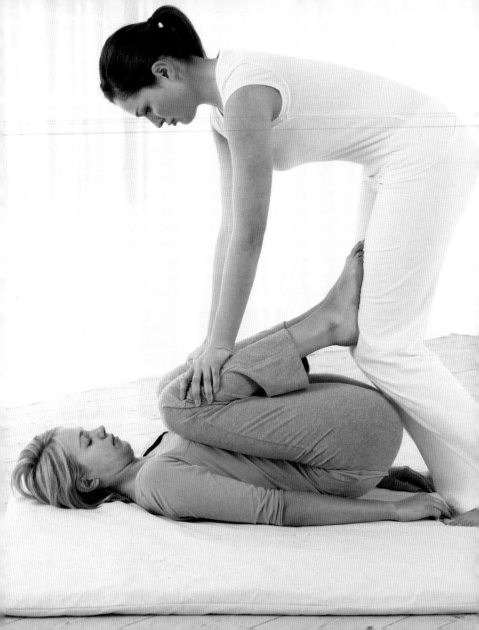

# Shiatsu

A Japanese therapy based on Chinese origins, the term *shiatsu* means simply "finger pressure." The following shiatsu sequence is based on relaxing the body and promoting the flow of energy (*ki*) and provides a general constitutional tonic. Applying the movements with sensitivity is better than using a checklist of techniques. The focus is on pressure and stretching to balance the meridians. The massage should be balanced and thoughtful and the mind calm, with a sense of connection between both partners. Where you feel any tension, try to ease it gently according to shiatsu principles or work on another related area.

# Principles

Developing as it has done from Chinese theory and principles of medicine, shiatsu shows numerous similarities with *TuiNa*. The application of shiatsu also depends on the flow of energy (*ki*) through channels known as meridians, although there are some differences from the Chinese acupressure model.

## The meridians

There are 12 pairs of meridians governed by, and retaining the characteristics of, the organs of the body, in addition to two central channels that are not related to specific organs. These two channels are known as the Governor and Conception Vessels (or Du and Ren), and are located at the back and front of the body respectively. *Yang* energy descends at the back and *yin* energy rises up the front of the body.

The balance of energy between the meridians and the relationship between individual and environment are of significance. As in Chinese philosophy, the five elements of water, fire, wood, metal, and earth are attributed to all aspects of life, and the balance between them produces conditions that can affect our state of health. The interplay between *yin* and *yang* is also crucial to achieving good health; *yin* (which is dark, female, and cool) and *yang* (light,

male, and hot) can also absorb and change into one another.

Originally practiced as a home remedy instead of acupuncture, shiatsu aims to promote the free flow of *ki* along the channels and to balance the various elements within the body. When they are out of balance, we are not only more vulnerable to disease, but disease is seen as a symptom of that lack of balance.

# The meridians (front)

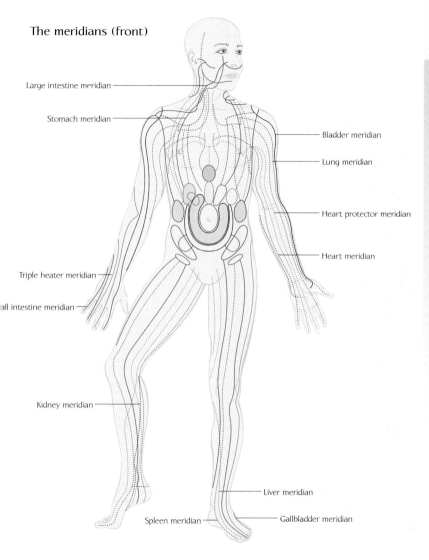

Large intestine meridian

Stomach meridian

Bladder meridian

Lung meridian

Heart protector meridian

Heart meridian

Triple heater meridian

all intestine meridian

Kidney meridian

Liver meridian

Spleen meridian

Gallbladder meridian

# The *tsubos*

Various pressure points are located along the meridians and are known in shiatsu as *tsubos*. There are 365 of them within the body; they are like communication centers and are generally located in weaker areas of the body or actual physical depressions.

Imbalances may be signified by changes in the surrounding muscle or skin. By applying pressure to the *tsubos* it is possible to correct imbalances within a meridian.

At any point along a meridian there may be an excess or deficiency of *ki*. Where there is an excess, the energy is described as *jitsu*. The area around this point may feel tense or hard, and pressure here may be sharp or painful; the condition may be acute. Where there is a deficiency of *ki*, the condition is described as *kyo*. The area around this point may feel soft or hollow, and pressure here may be more like an ache or can even be quite pleasurable; the condition is usually chronic.

Meridians are associated with the function of an organ, rather than simply with the organ itself. Treatment of any constriction takes the underlying cause into account, which may be due to a variety of factors. Physical symptoms may be linked to the internal environment, including constitutional energy and emotional factors, or to external influences that are depleting the individual.

It is possible to influence the energy of a point by working on another point further along the meridian in question; and to influence the energy of the meridian as a whole simply by working along its length. Professional treatment is often preceded by *hara* (abdomen) diagnosis (made by touching the abdomen with the hand) together with general observations that will determine the shiatsu sequence. Skill in feeling these differing states of energy comes with practice and experience, along with an understanding of how and where to apply pressure.

# The *tsubos* (front)

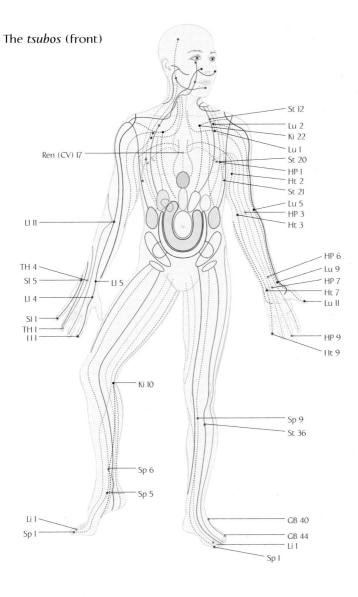

St 12
Lu 2
Ki 22
Lu 1
Ren (CV) 17
St 20
HP 1
Ht 2
St 21
Lu 5
HP 3
Ht 3
LI 11
HP 6
Lu 9
HP 7
Ht 7
Lu 11
TH 4
SI 5
LI 5
LI 4
SI 1
TH 1
LI 1
HP 9
Ht 9
Ki 10
Sp 9
St 36
Sp 6
Sp 5
Li 1
Sp 1
GB 40
GB 44
Li 1
Sp 1

# The *tsubos* (back)

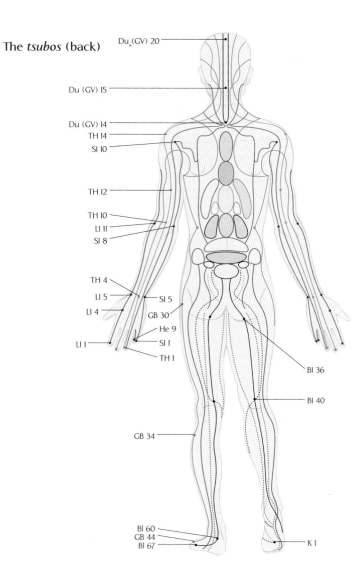

Du$_e$ (GV) 20

Du (GV) 15

Du (GV) 14
TH 14
SI 10

TH 12

TH 10
LI 11
SI 8

TH 4
LI 5
LI 4

SI 5
GB 30
He 9
SI 1
TH 1

LI 1

BI 36

BI 40

GB 34

BI 60
GB 44
BI 67

K 1

# The *tsubos* (head)

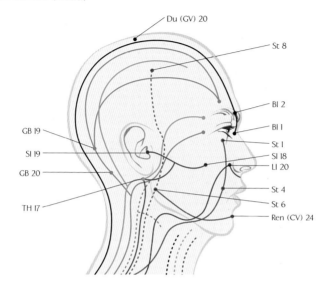

Du (GV) 20
St 8
Bl 2
Bl 1
GB 19
SI 19
GB 20
TH 17
St 1
SI 18
LI 20
St 4
St 6
Ren (CV) 24

# The *tsubos* (feet)

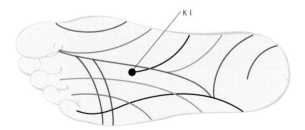

K 1

# Application

Shiatsu is traditionally applied fully clothed, with no creams or oil, with the receiver lying on the floor, although in Japan treatments are now often given on a massage table. The giver uses his or her body weight to apply pressure with the hands, as well as the elbows, forearms, knees, and feet.

Pressure should be slow and steady, the posture balanced and energy coming from the abdomen or *hara*. This provides physical as well as emotional stability. One hand, known as the "mother" hand, remains on the body for support. The limbs may be stretched or moved into various positions to provide more effective access to, and pressure on, the meridians. However, you must always take your own and your partner's flexibility into account.

Both giver and receiver should wear loose, comfortable clothing with adequate body support. Taking time to find comfortable positions is important. The giver needs to feel balanced, both physically and mentally, in order to lean in with their weight and give a good massage. Full, committed contact with each movement is vital, as is feedback from receiver to giver.

At the beginning, getting a sense of a person's energy is better than trying to

## FOCUS POINTS

**Techniques:** The main strokes are pressure with the fingers, thumbs, whole hand, elbows, and feet, with some rocking, rubbing, and stretches.

**Movements:** These should be slow and reassuring, balanced, and focused, using your whole body weight.

**Equipment:** You need a mat on the floor; and supports for the head, knees, or ankles.

**Feedback:** Check for any health problems first, and ask your partner for feedback.

**Timing:** A whole-body shiatsu treatment should take about 45 minutes.

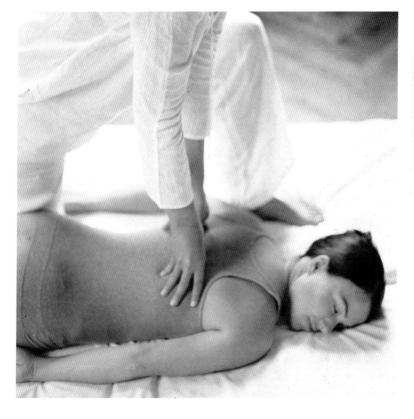

correct imbalances. Keep everything as simple as possible. In time you will learn how to detect a deficiency or excess of *ki* and the best way to go about applying a remedy. You will also begin to see beyond particular symptoms and take the bigger picture into account. In

*Shiatsu treatments are traditionally given on the floor. The giver then uses their body weight as they apply the movements.*

shiatsu, each person and their health is viewed as unique, so treatment is individual rather than formulaic.

# The back

Center yourself both emotionally and physically before beginning work on the back. You will need to be balanced and have enough room in order to apply the techniques. The back provides you with a good opportunity for exploring the use of your body weight.

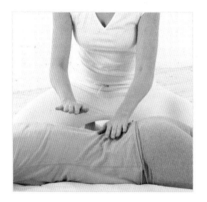

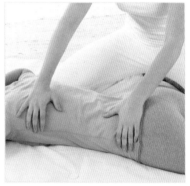

1 palm pressure Kneel to one side of your partner. Take a breath, lean forward and place both palms on the opposite side of the spine. "Walk" your hands up and down from the lower back to the shoulders, avoiding pressure on the spine. Lean your weight into your hands, but remain well balanced at all times. Repeat several times to relax your partner and increase your confidence.

2 rocking Positioned square on to your partner, place both hands over the muscles on the opposite side of the spine, over the bladder meridian. Rock the body away from you using the heels of your hands. Work several times up and down the meridian from lower back to shoulders, to relax the whole of the back.

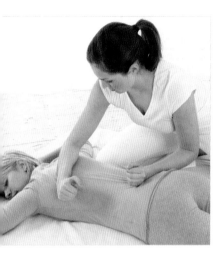

### 3 stretching with the forearms

Place your forearms together at a diagonal in the middle of the back. Your hands should form loose fists. Slowly stretch one arm over the back toward the shoulder, and the other toward the hip. Maintain full contact with your forearms so that your partner feels a good stretch. Without changing position, you can then repeat all the movements on the other side of the spine.

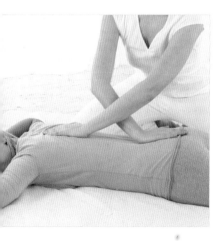

### 4 stretching with the palms

Kneel at the lower back. Cross your arms and place one hand over the sacrum (the bony triangle at the base of the spine) and the other further up the back. Without sliding them, push your hands away from each other to provide a stretch for the lower back. Check for resistance, then try again, this time stretching a little further.

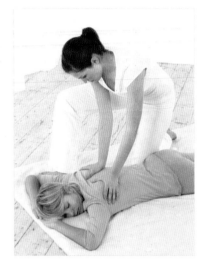

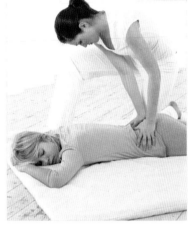

5 **palm pressure** Position yourself at your partner's upper back, with enough balance to lean across your partner. Center yourself at the *hara*. Place your palms flat on either side of the spine, with the heels on the muscles and your fingers pointing toward the ribs. Lean in toward the body and exert comfortable pressure. Work down to the lower back.

6 **palm pressure** Position yourself facing up the spine. Place your hands flat at either side of the lower back, with the heels facing inward and the fingers toward the hips. Press with the palms of both hands, using your body weight to exert pressure carefully. Check that this feels okay with your partner. Release the pressure evenly and lift your hands away.

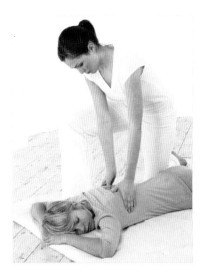
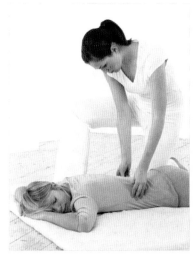

7 thumb pressure Return to the upper back. Place both thumbs over the muscles on either side of the spine, with the fingers providing support. Press with your thumbs along the bladder meridian down to the lower back. Press roughly in a line with the depressions between the vertebrae, always avoiding the spine. Use your body weight as necessary to slowly increase the pressure.

8 thumb pressure Place both thumbs at the lower back, about three finger-widths out from the spine. Locate the bands of muscle that become much broader here. Press in with your thumbs in three places to the sides of these muscles, along the outer bladder meridian. Press in, hold, then slowly release your pressure.

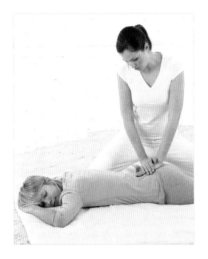

9 circling Move to your partner's lower back. Place both hands, one on top of the other, over the sacrum. Circle on the spot in a counterclockwise direction to relax the lower back and hips; this also helps to warm the kidneys. Repeat slowly and sensitively several times, molding your hands to the shape of the body.

10 rubbing Maintaining body contact with one hand, rub vigorously along the bladder meridian using the flats of your fingers. Rub from the shoulders down to the lower back along the inner meridian. Rub down the muscles of one side first, then repeat on the other side of the spine. End by placing one hand over the lower back, and rest for a few moments.

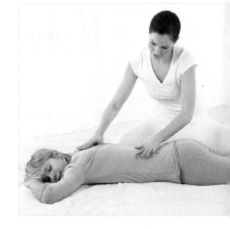

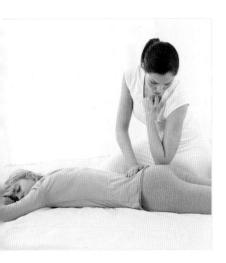

11 elbow pressure Using one hand for support over the lower back, lean into position with your elbow over your partner's buttock. Relax the angle of your elbow and let your hand flop at the wrist. Begin halfway across the buttock, and lean into the muscles with your elbow, then release. Work down the bladder channel to just above the buttock crease.

12 elbow pressure Locate GB 30, two-thirds of the way across the buttocks and one-third of the way down. Using your other hand for support, place your elbow—keeping it rounded—over the area and circle into the point. This is usually a tense but fleshy area, so you can use reasonable pressure. Keep continuous contact without sliding. Leaning across, repeat both movements on the opposite side.

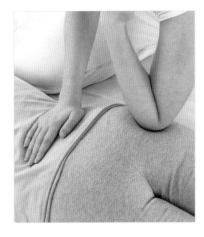

# Back of the legs and feet

Make sure that you are in a good position as you follow the leg sequence. The position of your partner's legs is also important as you apply pressure to the meridians. Careful pressure should be used over the joints. Make sure that you use similar pressure on both legs.

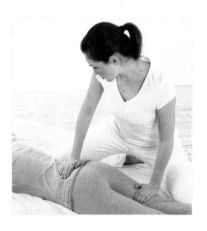 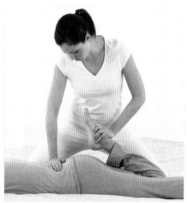

1 palm pressure Position yourself at your partner's hips. Placing one hand on the body for support, "walk" down the back of the leg along the bladder meridian with the palm of the other hand. Begin just below the buttocks and end above the ankle, with less pressure over the back of the knee. Position your hand, apply pressure, hold, then release gradually each time.

2 stretching With the leg in a central position, slide one hand under the ankle and bend the leg back toward the buttock, with one hand resting on the sacrum, at the base of the spine, for support. Being sensitive to your partner's flexibility, try and touch the heel to the buttock, but stop when you feel resistance. Release the stretch, relax, and try again.

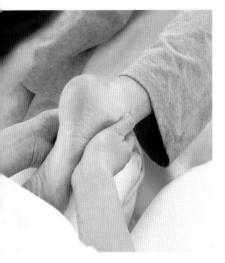

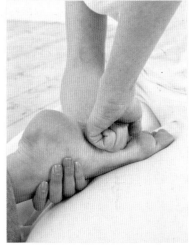

3 thumb circling Move to your partner's foot. Support it in your hands and circle both thumbs around the ankle bone to relax the joint. Work in as close to the ankle as possible and repeat several times. Press in with the balls of your thumbs and apply small circles on the spot to release blocked energy and stimulate the bloodflow to the feet.

4 kneading Knead over the ball of the foot with your knuckles, working around KI. Keep your hand as relaxed as possible to avoid digging in, with your other hand cradling underneath for resistance and support. You can extend the movements over the whole foot, but make sure that you avoid massaging over the instep.

CAUTION

Do not use point KI during pregnancy.

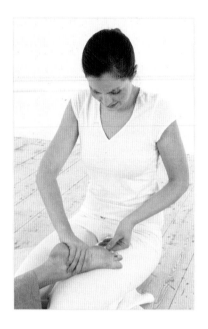

5 pulling Use your thumb, index, and middle fingers to pull each of the toes in turn. Squeeze down the outside of each toe, pull and give a little press, before ending contact. Extend the movement about 1 in. (2.5 cm) from the ends of the toes. Then lower the foot and repeat all the previous movements on the other leg.

6 pulling Kneel at your partner's feet. Slide both hands under the ankles, lift them slightly, then pull them toward you to provide a stretch. Take care not to overstrain yourself if your body weight is significantly less than your partner's. Repeat twice to release blocked energy from the joints.

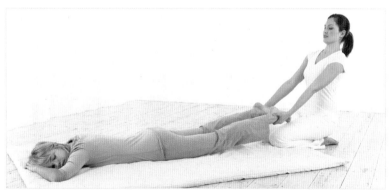

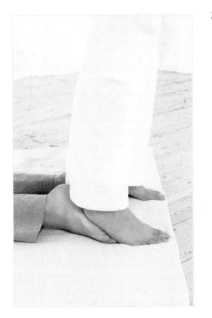

7 **foot pressure** Place your heels over the balls of your partner's feet, your toes resting on the floor. Apply pressure by gently "walking" up and down with your feet. Adjust your weight if necessary so that you apply pressure comfortably and evenly on the spot. Be careful to avoid any pressure over the instep.

8 **palm pressure** Ask your partner to turn on their side, upper leg bent toward the floor to expose the gallbladder meridian. Use a cushion for support under the knee. With one hand on the body for support, "walk" down the outside of the leg to the ankle, avoiding pressure at the knee. Contact is with the whole hand, pressure with the palm. Position, press, hold, and release, then repeat on the other leg.

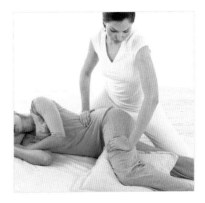

# The abdomen

Shiatsu over the *hara* or abdomen is sometimes given as a complete massage and is very important in professional diagnosis. Relaxation is key here. Use sensitivity, especially during menstruation when you might prefer to simply use the first step. Hara massage should be avoided during pregnancy.

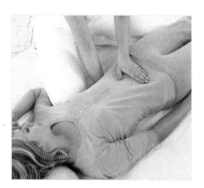

1 resting Place one hand under the back for support and the other flat on the abdomen, just below the navel. Keep your hands in contact as your partner breathes in and out, allowing your hands to rise and fall with the breath. Breathe calmly yourself, relax and put any thoughts to one side.

2 palm pressure With one hand on the abdomen for support, slowly apply pressure over the abdomen moving in a clockwise circle around the navel. Your hand should feel relaxing and reassuring. Be aware of any areas of tension. The pressure will have an effect on the inner organs and create a feeling of relaxation and well-being.

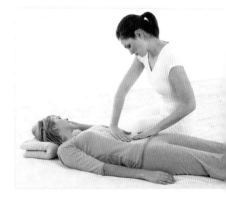

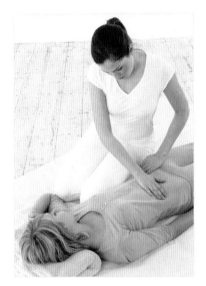

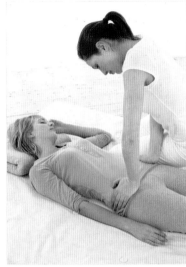

3 palm pressure Circle both hands over the abdomen to relax your partner. The direction should be clockwise around the navel, once again paying attention to any tense areas. Make sure one hand remains in contact with the body at all times for continuity and reassurance, and repeat the movements several times.

4 heel pressure Place your hands over your partner's hips, heels inward, fingers pointing to the floor. Very gently and slowly lean your weight into your palms, hold, then release the pressure. The movement should come from your *hara*. This helps to relax and open up the pelvic area, but great care should be taken not to press too hard.

# The chest

Work from a balanced position over the chest, so that you can easily regulate your pressure. Avoid applying any pressure directly on the breasts. From here the sequence continues in a clockwise direction around your partner's body until you once again return to the chest.

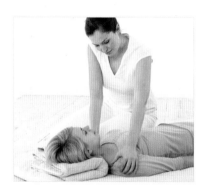

1 palm pressure Lean over your partner, but retain control of your balance. Place the heels of both hands over the ribcage, just beneath the balls of the shoulders, with your fingers facing toward the arms. Lean into your hands and apply pressure evenly with your palms. Lean back again as you release the pressure.

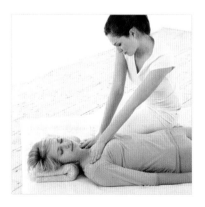

2 palm pressure Move your hands so that the palms are over the ribcage on either side of the sternum, just above the breasts. The heels of your hands should be facing each other, with the fingers pointing away. Lean into your hands to apply steady pressure, hold for a moment, then lean back as you release. This stimulates LU 2.

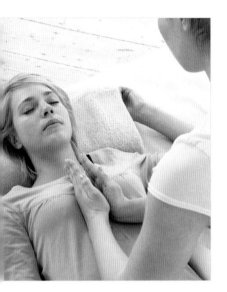

3 **finger pressure** Place both hands facing each other just below the collarbone, about 1 in. (2.5 cm) either side of the sternum. Apply pressure over the ribs, working down the center of the body toward the diaphragm. This is a simple way to avoid heavy pressure as well as any pressure over the breasts.

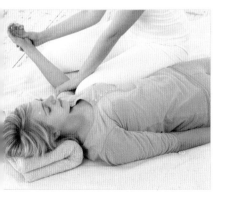

4 **passive rotation** Bring your partner's arm out to the side. With one hand steadying the arm at the elbow, grasp the hand in your own and lift the forearm. From here slowly rotate the arm at the elbow in both directions. This helps to relax the joints and improve the flow of energy through the meridians.

# The arms and hands

Begin the sequence on the arm nearest to you, including a stretch, and work right down to the tips of the fingers for a final release of energy. From here the sequence continues around the body so you will complete work on the opposite arm when you have reached the other side.

1 **palm pressure** Position yourself at your partner's side. Place the arm, palm facing upward, at a right angle to the body. With one hand resting on the shoulder for support, apply pressure with your other palm along the inner arm, working from the shoulder to the wrist. Check your balance, position your palm, lean in with your weight, and then release evenly and steadily.

2 **thumb pressure** Locate HP 6, which is in the middle of the forearm, about two and a half finger-widths up from the wrist. Keep contact with your partner's arm with one hand and place your thumb over the point. Press in slowly and steadily with the ball of your thumb, then release equally steadily. This is a good point for stress relief. Repeat several times.

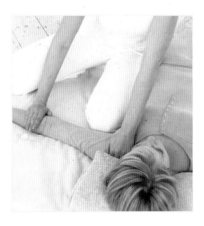

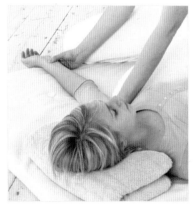

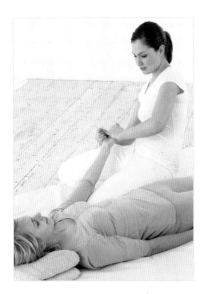

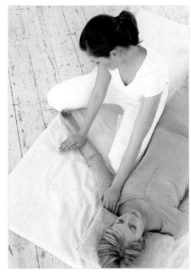

3 pulling Grasp your partner's hand
securely, lift the arm and pull back
toward you to give a stretch. Your
position should be balanced so that
you can use your body weight and
imagine the movement coming from
your *hara*. The stretch helps to release
any energy around the joints.

4 heel pressure With one hand on
the shoulder for support, use the heel
of your other hand to press along the
inner arm, following the lung meridian.
Place your hand, press, hold, and release
at regular intervals working your way
to the hand. Press over the thumb and
squeeze the tip for a final release.

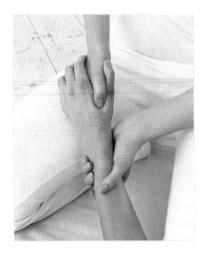

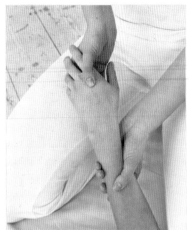

5 **thumb pressure** Locate LI 4, which lies in the web of the hand between the index finger and thumb. Place your thumb in position, circle over the spot, then press it between your finger and the tip of your thumb. Hold for a few moments, then release your pressure. For a more subtle effect, simply circle on the spot with the ball of your thumb.

6 **squeezing** Place your third finger and thumb in the web of your partner's hand between their index finger and thumb. Reach as high as you can, then squeeze as you pull between the tendons and bones to the fingers. As you do so, jiggle between the thumb and finger so that you get a zigzag effect. Repeat between the tendons across the back of the hand.

### CAUTION

Do not use point LI 4 during pregnancy.

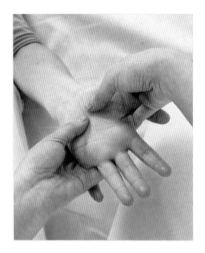
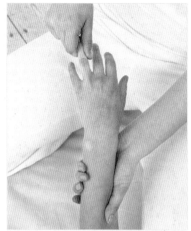

7 **thumb pressure** Turn the hand so that the palm faces upward, interlace your little fingers and support from underneath. This stretches out the fingers and helps to open up the palm. Then press fairly firmly over the surface with both thumbs to stimulate as much of the hand as possible.

8 **squeezing** Grasp your partner's thumb between your own thumb and fingers and squeeze down to the tip. Twist along the side of the thumb, pressing quite firmly, squeeze at the nailbed, then pull off the thumb with a flick. Repeat the movements over each finger in turn. This helps to both stimulate and release energy.

# Front of the legs and feet

The sequence now works up the front of the body following the meridians. Take care as you move the legs into position to keep within your partner's comfort zone. The pressure you use should be similar for both legs, with gentle pressure applied to the joints.

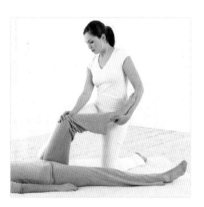

1  passive rotation Move to your partner's foot. Slip one hand under the ankle and the other under the knee and carefully raise the leg. Use your body weight to gently rotate the leg at the hip, your own leg providing support where necessary. Rotate several times in both directions to relax the hip then carefully lower the leg to the floor.

2  palm pressure Position yourself at your partner's thigh. Keep contact with one hand on the abdomen, and use the other hand to "walk" down the side of the thigh to the knee to stimulate the stomach meridian. Position, press, hold, and release. Continue carefully over the knee and down the side of the lower leg. Lift your hand when you reach the ankle and repeat several times.

3 **thumb pressure** Locate St 36 by running your thumb along the line of the shinbone until you come to the curve of the bone just below the knee. Hold your thumb in position, then press slowly with the ball of the thumb. Check the pressure with your partner because this point can often be sensitive. St 36 is a good tonic point for the digestive system.

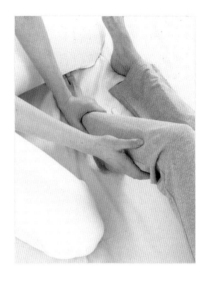

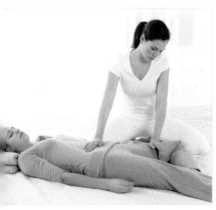

4 **palm pressure** Place your hands underneath the knee and the foot. Bend the leg and bring it out to the side. Keeping contact with the abdomen, "walk" down the inside of the leg with the palm of the other hand. This stimulates the liver meridian. Adjust your movements to your partner's flexibility and use a cushion for support if necessary. Apply a gentler pressure over the knee. Repeat several times.

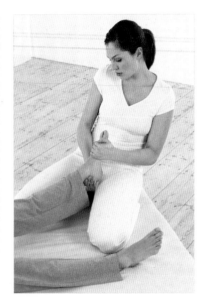

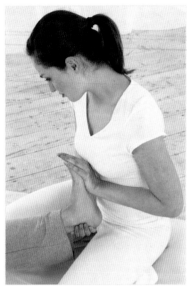

5 pulling Making sure your own position is steady, slide one hand under the ankle and the other over the top of the foot. Raise the leg slightly then pull back toward you to provide a stretch. Relax then try again. This is good for releasing energy from the joints and helping the flow of energy to and from the feet.

6 palm pressure Cradling the ankle in one hand for support, place your palm over the ball of your partner's foot. Press the foot back toward your partner, helping to release the ankle joint. The range of movement will depend on your partner's flexibility, but repeat several times, each time pushing a little further to provide a stretch at the back of the leg.

7 **pushing** With your feet shoulder width apart, knees bent and in a balanced position, lift both your partner's legs at once and place the soles of the feet against your thighs. Lean forward and push against your partner, as if you were trying to push them away from you. Using the resistance of their body weight, this movement helps to relax and balance the body.

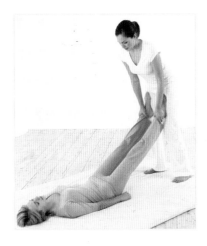

8 **passive rotation** From this position lean further forward, reach below your partner's knees and bend the legs toward the chest, using your body weight to increase the stretch. You can then rotate both legs at once in both directions to relax the lower back. Lower the legs carefully then repeat the preceding sequences on the other leg.

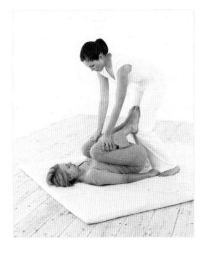

# The neck and scalp

Before beginning work on the neck and scalp you need to complete the shiatsu sequence on your partner's other arm. With the body now relaxed the neck massage should be easier for your partner. Encourage their trust by cradling their head with confidence. This will help them to really let go.

1 pulling Having completed the arm sequence on pages 224–227, position yourself at your partner's head. Lean forward, grasp both arms at the wrist then lean back with your body weight to provide a stretch to the arms and torso. Hold for several moments, checking comfort levels with your partner, then slowly release and guide the arms back down to the floor.

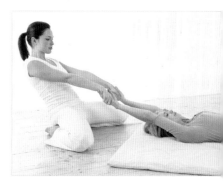

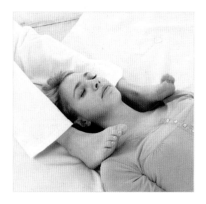

2 foot pressure Sitting behind your partner, knees slightly bent, place both your heels over the tops of your partner's shoulders. Place your hands behind you on the floor to steady you, then push each shoulder away from you in turn. Repeat gently several times to relax the shoulders and spine. Your partner should relax so their body rocks with the movement.

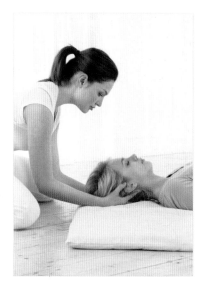

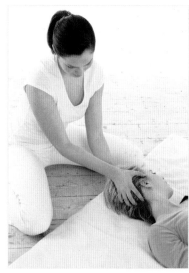

3 pulling Slide both hands under the neck and position them at the base of the skull, so that the head is cradled in your hands. Lift the head slightly and give a stretch by pulling it toward you, sitting back on your heels as you do so. Keeping your arms outstretched enables you to remain well balanced. Slide your hands right under the skull and lower the head again gently.

4 rocking Cradling the base of your partner's skull in your hands, gently turn the head from side to side. This relaxes the neck muscles. Start slowly, then as your partner relaxes you can use a gentle rocking movement. Encourage your partner to let go so that you perform the movements without either their resistance or help.

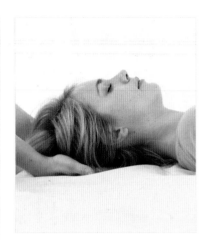

5 finger pressure Using the tip of your middle finger as a guide, run it up the spine until you locate the depression just below the base of your partner's skull. Once in position, press gently in toward GV 15 with the ball of your finger, hold for a moment and then release. This is very good for promoting calm.

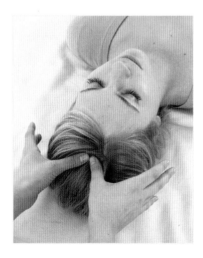

6 thumb pressure Cup your hands around the head, with your thumbs together at the hairline. Apply pressure with the balls of both thumbs together, working back in a central line over the scalp. Follow the rhythm of locating, pressing, holding, and releasing, so that your movements and pressure are applied evenly and smoothly.

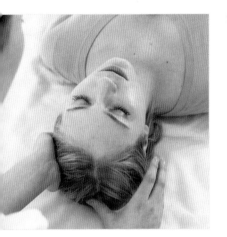

7 **thumb pressure** When you reach the midpoint, in a line up from the middle of the ears, you will be able to feel a slight depression. At this point press in very slowly toward Du (GV) 20 with the ball of your thumb. Circle minutely on the spot. This is very good for lifting the spirits and generally releasing tension.

8 **percussion** For scalp stimulation, press down on the scalp with the fingers and thumbs of both hands, then remove them suddenly so that your fingers almost bounce off the scalp. Use the balls of your fingers and keep your movements quick and light. End by tugging the hair gently.

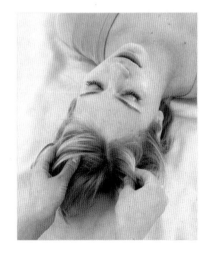

# The face

This face massage needs to be precise, both in order to feel good and for effective point stimulation. It is an uplifting way to end the massage, at once both deeply relaxing and energizing. The final resting stroke provides balance and alignment before the massage ends.

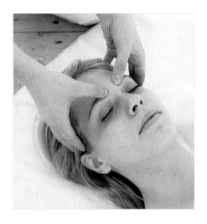

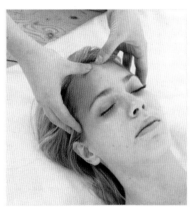

1 **thumb pressure** Place both thumbs on your partner's eyebrows, just beside the bridge of the nose. Locate Bl 2 by finding the small depressions in the bone. Press with the sides of the tips of your thumbs, as this point needs to be precise. Hold for a few moments, then release. Press sensitively because these points are often tender.

2 **thumb pressure** Press with the balls of your thumbs in a line up from the inner line of the eyebrows to the hairline. This movement should be slow, steady and relaxing and should follow the bladder meridian. Repeat the lines over the forehead several times.

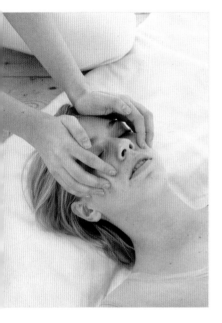

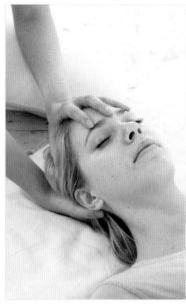

3 finger pressure Press with the tips of your fingers in a line under the cheekbones, working out toward the angle of the jaw. Press close to, and slightly upward under, the bone, keeping your pressure and the movements light.

4 resting Cradle your hand under the base of your partner's skull and place the other over the forehead. Pull very slightly toward you to align the head then simply rest. Empty any thoughts from your mind and breathe calmly. This provides a quiet moment before the massage ends and tells your partner the sequence is complete.

# Shiatsu quick fix

This shortened version of the shiatsu massage contains some of the most important steps. Perform each one with equal attention and focus, for the best effect. In keeping with the full length massage, keep changes in body position to a minimum.

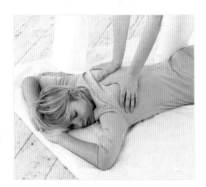

1 palm pressure on the back

Position the heels of both hands between your partner's shoulder blades, on either side of the spine. Your fingers should point toward the sides of the body. Lean into your hands to apply pressure on the muscles and stimulate the bladder meridian. Work at an even pace right down to the lower back.

2 elbow pressure on the hips

Round your elbow, place it on the buttock and locate GB 30, two-thirds of the way across and one-third of the way down. Apply reasonable pressure toward the body. Continue pressing over and around the hip. Repeat on the other side or, if you feel confident, try pressing both elbows into the buttocks at once.

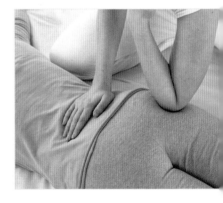

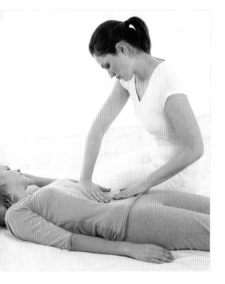

3 **palm pressure on the abdomen** Place one hand on the body for support while you press around the navel in a clockwise direction with the other. Keep your palm flat and feel for any areas of tension. Doing this in a regulated, relaxed way encourages tension release which will in turn lead to deeper, fuller breathing.

4 **pulling the neck** Sit at the head. Slide your hands under the neck until you can cradle the base of the skull in your hands. Make sure that your partner is relaxed before you lean back with your body weight, pulling gently toward you to provide a stretch. Slide your hands right under the back of the head to lower it again.

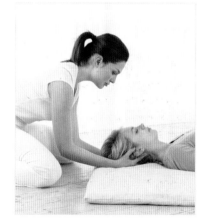

# Self-massage

During the following self-massage the techniques that you have applied to a partner can be used for massage on yourself. You can either try them while sitting on the floor, or on a chair if that feels more comfortable. Set aside a few minutes when you can concentrate fully on your own body and mind.

1 percussion on the upper back

Make a loose fist, then pummel up and down the muscles along the top of your opposite shoulder. Work from the neck toward the arm and back again several times. Your movements should be stimulating and over the fleshy muscle, rather than bone. This will stimulate the bladder and gallbladder meridians. Repeat over your opposite shoulder.

2 finger pressure on the neck

Reach behind your head and locate GV 15, which lies in a central position just beneath the base of your skull. Press with your fingers, pressing up and under the skull. Hold for a few moments. You will know when you have got the right point because you will feel the energy resonate, which produces a physical reaction. This point is good for relaxation.

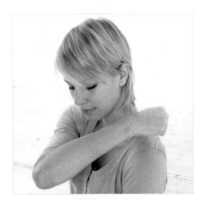

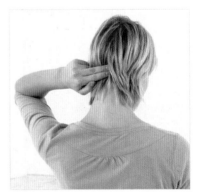

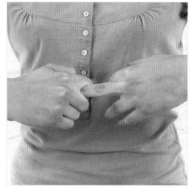

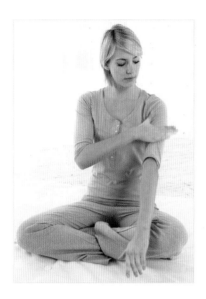

3 rubbing the arms With the flat of your hand, reach over and rub briskly up the outside of your arm from wrist to shoulder, rubbing in several lines. Then turn the palm over and rub down the inner arm to stimulate the circulation. This will help if you have cold hands. Repeat on the other arm.

4 pulling the fingers Grasp the fingers of one hand by bending the index and middle fingers of the other. This way you can grasp, squeeze, and pull each finger and the thumb in turn. Begin at the base of the fingers and pull firmly down to the tips. This releases energy through the hand. Repeat on your other hand.

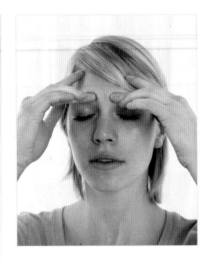

## 5 finger pressure on the face

Place your middle fingers just by the inner line of your eyebrows. You will feel a small depression in the bone. Press directly into the point with the tips of the fingers—it may feel a little sensitive. This is Bl 2 and is very good for sinus headaches. Hold for a few moments, then release.

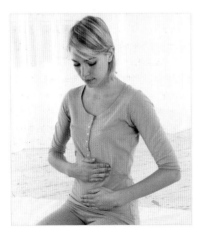

## 6 palm pressure on the abdomen

Breathe calmly, center yourself and place both hands flat on the abdomen. Circle gently in a clockwise direction around the navel, pausing at intervals to press your abdomen with your palms. This helps to stimulate the intestines. Repeat slowly several times.

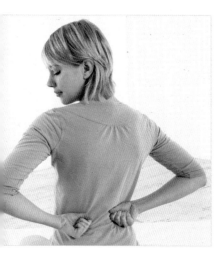

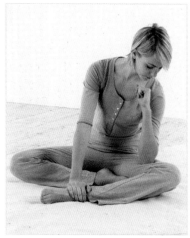

7 **knuckle pressure on the back**

Form your hands into loose fists and reach up behind your back. Place your hands on the muscle bands to the sides of your spine in line with your kidneys. Slowly circle your knuckles over the muscles, the direction is in toward your spine. This stimulates the kidneys while relaxing the lower back.

8 **elbow pressure on the legs**

Sitting cross-legged on the floor, round your elbow and press along the inside of your thigh at regular intervals to stimulate both the liver and spleen meridians. With the leg bent out the meridians are exposed but this can also be done sitting on a chair. Press and release at an even pace over both legs.

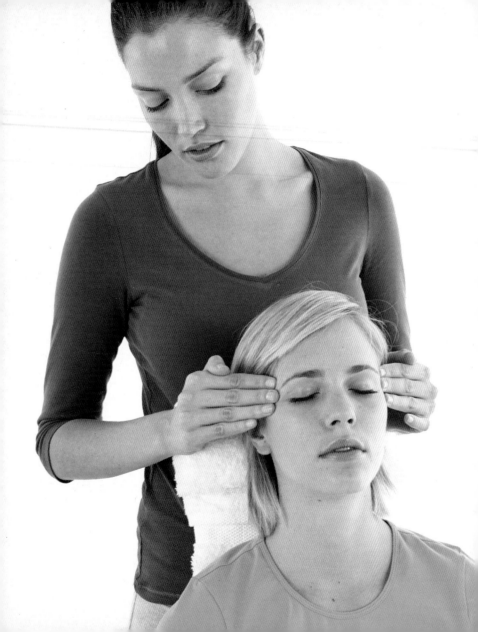

# Indian head massage

Indian head massage is an energizing upper body treatment. While stimulating techniques are used, it needs to be performed with sensitivity over the neck and head. The massage relaxes the muscles using a number of swift percussion movements, and ends by stimulating the scalp, with the option of using nourishing oils over the hair. The giver needs to maintain a balanced posture and concentrate on keeping a straight spine. The energy exchange between both participants is a vital ingredient of this form of massage.

# Principles

The term Ayurveda comes from the Sanskrit word meaning "science of life" and is the complex ancient system of philosophy and medicine in which Indian head massage has its roots. Ayurveda considers balance and moderation to be essential for health, with body and mind being inextricably linked.

According to Ayurvedic thought, the universe is made up of five elements—ether, air, earth, fire, and water—and human beings are made up of a combination of these elements.

## The *doshas*

In addition, there are believed to be three *doshas*, or energies, that exist in all matter. These are called *vata*, *pitta*, and *kapha*. Most people have one dominant *dosha*, and an Ayurvedic treatment will take this into consideration. *Vata* is the air energy, and these types tend to be thin, restless, anxious, creative, and have dry skin. *Pitta* is a mixture of fire and water energy, and these types are active, decisive, with a good appetite, thin hair, and smooth skin; they also sweat easily. *Kapha* is a mixture of water and earth energy, and these types tend to be overweight, move slowly, sleep a lot, and have thick hair and oily skin.

## The *chakras*

The vital energy that moves through the body is referred to as *prana*. There are seven main energy circles, or *chakras*, located along the spine through which *prana* flows. These *chakras* generate energy that is transmitted to smaller centers within the body. The first six *chakras* are located in the genital, sacral, solar-plexus, heart, neck, and forehead areas; the seventh is located at the top of the head. When the energy flowing through the *chakras* becomes blocked, this results in mental and physical disorders. Ayurvedic massage encourages the free flow of energy and as a result promotes good health.

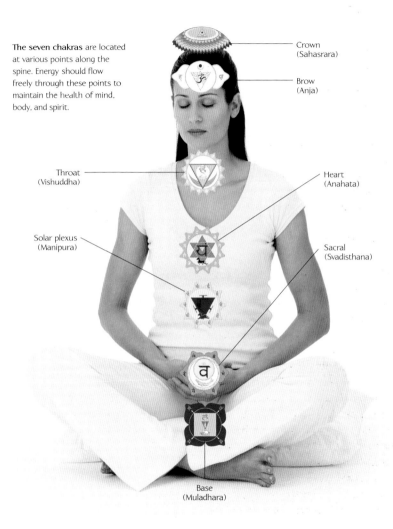

**The seven chakras** are located at various points along the spine. Energy should flow freely through these points to maintain the health of mind, body, and spirit.

Crown
(Sahasrara)

Brow
(Anja)

Throat
(Vishuddha)

Heart
(Anahata)

Solar plexus
(Manipura)

Sacral
(Svadisthana)

Base
(Muladhara)

# *Marma* points

The *chakras* are thought to correspond to the *marmas*, to which they transmit vital energy or *prana*. There are three main *marma* centers, located in the head, heart, and bladder which are vital to our health and survival. The body's vital force can be influenced by massaging *marma* points.

*Marma* points are points of energy distributed throughout the body, and there are 107 of them (including the five regions of the skull). They contribute to our health by stimulating organ function and maintaining equilibrium. The *marma* points are areas of concentrated energy, referred to as secret or hidden, and they provide a connection between our physical and subtle energies. They are mostly located at the meeting point between body systems and in areas such as the arteries, veins, tendons, and joints. Each point corresponds to a particular *dosha* (see pages 246–247) and has a related physical symptom. When these points are blocked we become ill.

The free flow of energy through the *chakras* can be facilitated by gentle massage of the *marma* points—or marmapuncture, which is similar to acupuncture. This massage unblocks energy, helps eliminate illness, and restores the body to health. *Marma* massage uses a variety of oils that contain different qualities: they may be calming, cooling, or burning and are related to the three *doshas* (see pages 246–247). The oil that is used will depend on the *dosha* type of the receiver and the imbalance that is being treated. Essential oils may also sometimes be used on the points by a skilled practitioner.

Indian head massage stimulates the *marma* points of the upper body, face, and head and helps to balance the energy in the higher *chakras*.

# The marma points

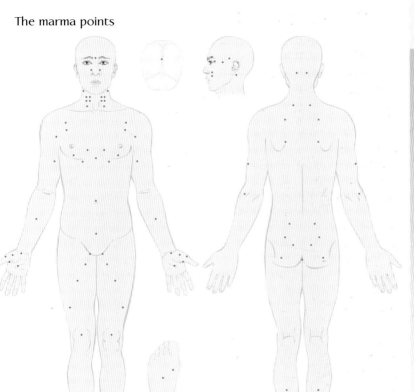

# Application

Indian head massage takes place seated, through clothes. First the upper back is relaxed—which is where most people store a lot of tension—before working over the neck and head. The strokes are fairly brisk and vigorous, stimulating the nervous system as well as energy points and channels.

Indian head massage is also known as champissage, from which the word "shampoo" is derived. It has been practiced in families in Asia for more than a thousand years and forms part of a grooming and beauty ritual. Indian head massage helps to relax the muscles, improves the circulation (particularly to the scalp, where it can promote healthy hair growth), and promotes lymph flow. It can help to relieve tension headaches, sinus problems, eyestrain, and even jaw problems related to tension. The massage works on the three upper *chakras* and can induce calmness and mental relaxation. Oils may (but need not be) used over the scalp, and should be left on the hair for several hours afterward; they should only be used in the last phase of the massage. The posture of the receiver should be upright, but relaxed, and a seat with a low back is ideal.

## FOCUS POINTS

Techniques: The main strokes are percussion, rotating, rubbing, finger pressure, and sawing.

Movements: These are vigorous and energizing, yet sensitive to energy, maintaining a good balanced posture, and using the body weight.

Equipment: You need a seat with a low back; a small cushion or towel for support; and some oil for the hair if you choose to use this.

Feedback: Check for any health problems first (particularly any neck problems) and ask your partner for feedback, because the techniques are relatively vigorous.

Timing: An Indian head massage should take about 30 minutes.

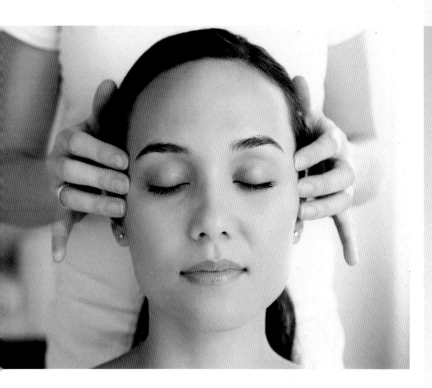

The beauty of Indian head massage is that it can be performed almost anywhere and is completed in about two-thirds the time of a full body massage. While it is stimulating, the effect is a complete sense of well-being, balance and calm. However, be

*A traditional Indian head massage energizes the upper body, relieves tension, and promotes a healthy heart.*

especially careful where there are any neck problems and, if in doubt, seek professional advice.

# The upper back

The massage begins on the upper back and progressively relaxes the body as you move up toward the head. Keep an eye on your own posture and make your movements brisk and dynamic. Once the back is relaxed, half your work is done!

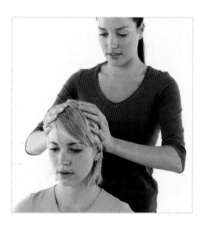

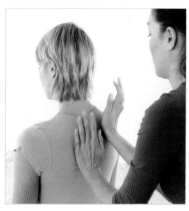

1 first touch Stand behind your partner and suggest some relaxed, slow breaths. Breathe deeply yourself and make sure that your posture is well balanced, with both feet planted evenly on the ground. Take a breath in and, as you breathe out, place your hands slowly on the crown of your partner's head. Relax, hold for a few moments, then withdraw your hands.

2 rubbing Rub briskly over your partner's back with the flats of your hands, one on either side of the spine. Begin just by the shoulders, then spread out and fan up and down the sides of the spine. This helps to stimulate the muscles and prepares the back for massage. Contact at this stage is on the surface rather than deep.

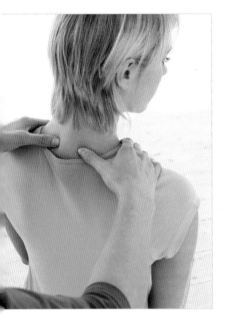

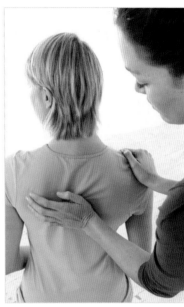

3  circling Place your thumbs on either
side of the spine, with your fingers
resting over the tops of the shoulders.
Locate the prominent vertebra, C7, at
the top of the spine and circle around
the area with your thumbs. Avoid any
pressure on the spine itself. You can
use fairly firm pressure here as long as
it feels comfortable.

4  heel pressure Stand to one side
and place the heel of your hand
between the shoulder blade and the
spine. Use your other hand to support
the body. Rub briskly over the muscles
and apply as much pressure as feels
good. Note that when these muscles
are tense, they can be quite sensitive.
Repeat on the other side.

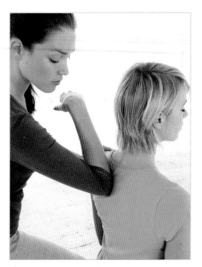

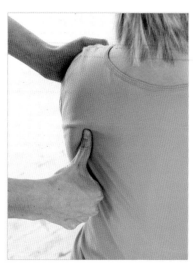

5 **elbow pressure** Stand to one side of your partner. Locate the vertebra in line with the top of the shoulder blade. Using your finger as a guide, support and modifier of pressure, relax your elbow, and press between the ribs, working about 1 in. (2.5 cm) out from the spine. Keep your elbow rounded so that the movement does not jab, and continue until you are level with the bottom of the blade. Repeat on the other side.

6 **thumb pressure** Keeping one hand on the body for support, locate the outline of the shoulder blade. Press between the ribs with the ball of your thumb, beginning level with the top of the blade. Press in four equal spaces around the shoulder. Keep the movements close in to the bone and repeat the sequence on the other side.

7 percussion Stand behind your partner. Keeping both hands relaxed, place your palms facing each other over one shoulder. Hack over the top of the shoulder from the neck toward the arm and back several times. The movements should be like chopping alternately with your hands, and need to be light, sharp, and quick. Repeat on the other shoulder.

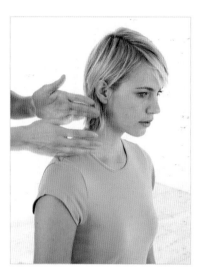

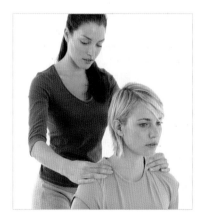

8 squeezing Place both hands over the tops of the shoulders, with your thumbs facing the spine and your fingers curled over the collarbone. Feel the line of fleshy muscle along the top of the shoulders. Lift and squeeze between the thumbs and fingers. Take care that the movements do not pinch, and work out toward the arms from the neck.

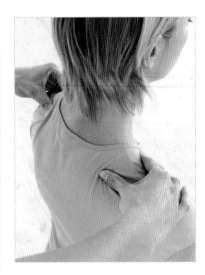

9 kneading Knead and squeeze along the tops of your partner's shoulders, rolling over the muscles with your fingers and thumbs. Press in with your thumbs and squeeze the muscles as you roll your fingers back toward you. Work across the shoulders with both hands at once, from the neck toward the arms, then back again.

10 pummelling Form both hands into loose fists and begin pummelling over one shoulder. Work from the arm toward the neck, then down one side of the spine to the lower back. Your movements should be brisk and quick, pummelling with the fists alternately. Work up and down the muscles alongside the spine several times, then cross to the other shoulder and repeat.

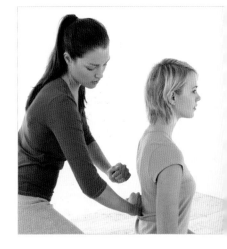

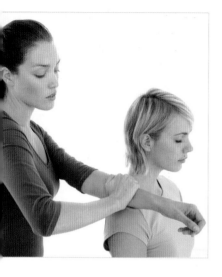

## 11 stretching with the forearms

Stand to one side. Lean forward with your spine straight, and place your forearm over the muscles at the top of the shoulder. Lean your weight forward again and apply pressure with your forearm, pressing with your other hand at the wrist to guide the movement. Press in three equal spaces between the neck and shoulder, then repeat on the other side.

## 12 stretching with the forearms

Lean with the backs of your forearms over the shoulder muscles, applying pressure and drawing them out across the shoulders toward the arms. This helps to relax the upper back as well as connect to the next sequence. Do this several times, ending by rolling your forearms to continue the movement down the upper arms.

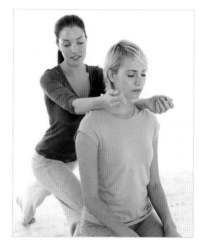

# The arms

Work on the arms follows on from the shoulder sequence and helps to relax the upper body. Ensure that you can move around your partner easily, and bend your knees so that you can reach comfortably rather than having to stoop over them.

1 effleurage With your partner's arms relaxed, stroke down the upper arms. This is an effleurage stroke done without oil. Mold your hands to the shape of the arms and stroke as far as the elbows. Repeat several times, then repeat over the back of the arms to help relax the muscles.

2 rubbing Repeat the same movements down the outer arms with a brisk rubbing movement, using the flats of your hands. Rub down the arms to the elbows, as before. Your spine should remain as straight as possible, and you should bend at the knees rather than leaning over your partner. Repeat briskly several times.

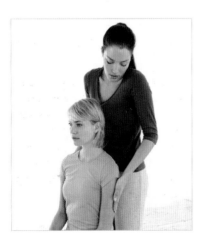

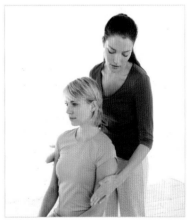

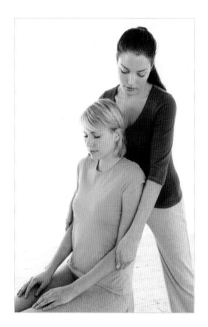

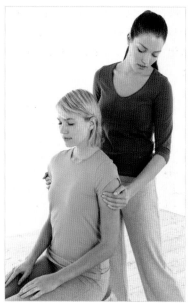

3 lifting Reach forward and cradle your partner's elbows in your hands so that the arms feel secure. Raise both elbows at the same time so that the shoulders hunch, but do not force or strain them. Keep your hands close to the body to protect the elbows. Hold for a few moments, then release and your partner's shoulders should relax and drop down.

4 squeezing Curl your fingers around the upper arms, using full hand contact with the heels and the palms. Squeeze the muscles between your fingers and heels, being careful not to pinch the skin. Squeeze down the arms at equal distances from shoulder to elbow, then repeat several times.

# The neck

A lot of tension tends to center in the neck. Encourage relaxation there by repetitive movements, and as you work on the neck reduce your pressure and speed. Support your partner's body as you massage so that the head does not drop forward.

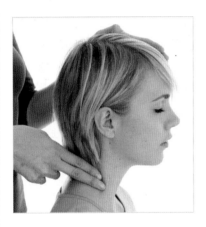

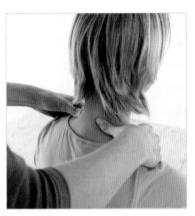

1 sawing Use your index and middle fingers together for this movement. Place them on the crest of the muscles at the top of your partner's shoulder. Begin a sawing movement back and forth over the muscles to relax them. Check the pressure with your partner. Continue sawing at equal distances along the shoulder and carefully up the neck. Repeat on the other side.

2 circling Place both thumbs on the muscles at the base of the neck, about 1 in. (2.5 cm) out from the spine on either side. With your fingers sitting on the shoulders for support, begin circling over the muscles with your thumbs. The circles should be like spirals traveling up to the base of the skull. Repeat several times.

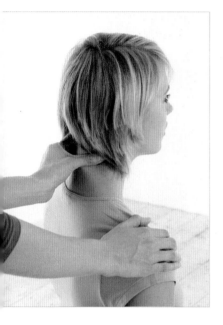

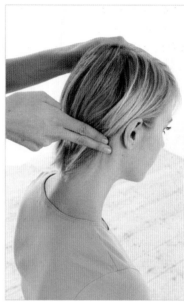

3 squeezing Place your hand at the back of the neck, with your thumb over the muscles on one side of the spine and your fingers over the muscles on the other side. Draw your hand back toward you, squeezing between fingers and thumb. Squeeze in several positions as far as the base of the skull. Change hands as you repeat the movement.

4 sawing Place your index and middle fingers together. Begin sawing lightly over the muscles at the base of the skull, moving towards the spine. Check that the pressure is okay with your partner, as the movements should be quite brisk. Stop 1 in. (2.5 cm) away from the spine, then repeat on the other side.

# The head

Working over the head is what makes this massage stand out. Use the techniques given below and repeat them as often as you like. Smooth the hair each time after ruffling it, and keep the head supported so that your partner can relax more easily.

1 rubbing Supporting your partner's head with one hand, rub over one side of the scalp with your other hand. Keep it flat and rub briskly over the hair. The movements should be quick and light and should cover as much of the head as possible. Change hands and repeat so that you cover the whole head with sufficient pressure to stimulate the scalp and boost the circulation.

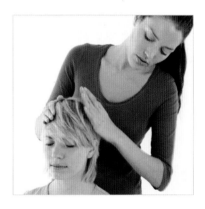

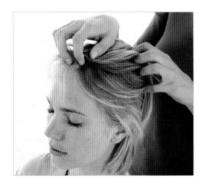

2 finger pressure Supporting the head with one hand, rake the fingers of your other hand through the hair. Use your fingertips to stimulate the scalp and to comb the hair away from the face. Make wave-like movements through the hair and over the scalp, always working toward the back of the head. Change hands to cover the whole scalp.

3 plucking Place your thumbs and fingertips on the scalp, then pull away with light plucking movements. One hand should follow the other, working over the head. As you pluck, lift the hair away from the scalp. The accent is on lifting and pulling away. This lightens the energy around the head.

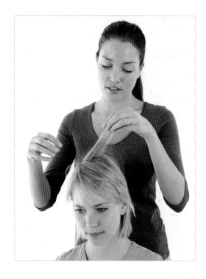

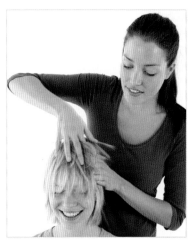

4 rubbing Smooth the hair and then, supporting the head with one hand, rub over the hairline with the other. Your fingers should point downward and move lightly over the scalp, creating a windscreen-wiper effect. Begin at the forehead and work to the back of the head, flicking the hair as much as possible. Change hands to cover the rest of the head.

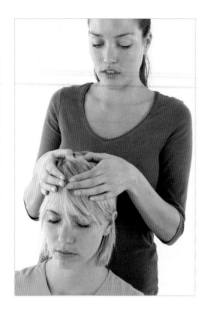

5 **thumb circling** Place both thumbs in the center of the scalp, with your fingers cupped around your partner's head. With the flats of your thumbs, circle in continuous spirals in a line to the back of the head. Change position to work back in a line a little further out, then repeat so that you cover as much of the head as possible. Make sure that you reach the back of the ears and circle around the hairline.

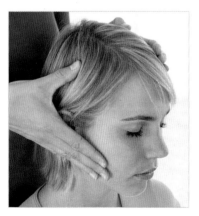

6 **thumb pressure** Hold the head firmly, then place your thumb and fingers on top of the head, and rotate over the scalp with your thumb. Work back in lines from the forehead, applying pressure on the spot each time. Cover as much of the scalp as you can, paying equal attention to the sides and back of the head.

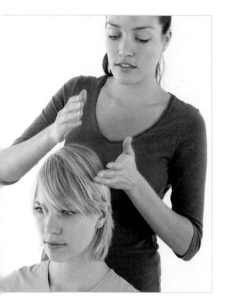

7 **percussion** Place both hands, palms facing each other, in position over the scalp. Keeping your hands relaxed, hack up and down over the head. The chopping movements should be quick and light. As your little fingers make brief contact with the scalp, you should create the typical snapping sound. The more relaxed your wrists are, the better your movements will be.

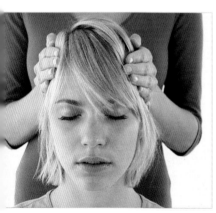

8 **squeezing** Place both hands, palms flat, just above the ears. Your fingers should face to the front, with the palms cupped around the head. Gently squeeze your hands together and lift slightly so that you move the scalp. Relax your hands without losing contact or changing position. Repeat the movement slowly twice more.

# The face

These strokes help to relax key points on the face to complete the relaxation process. Place the towel so that your partner feels secure—you should then be able to reach the points quite easily. Take extra care to keep your fingers away from the eyes.

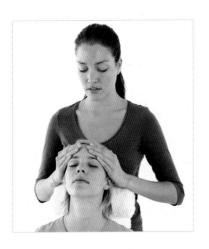

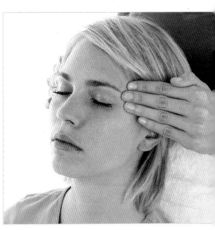

1 finger pressure Ask your partner to lean back against a small cushion or towel. Place your fingertips together in the center of the forehead and slowly draw your hands apart. It is best to press with the flats of your fingers. Imagine that you are drawing all the tension away from the forehead. Repeat several times.

2 circling Place your fingertips over the temples. Gently circle over the temples, rotating back toward you. The skin should move under your fingers. This helps to relax the mind and is good for relieving headaches. However, take great care not to press too firmly, and check with your partner that the level of pressure feels comfortable.

3 **finger pressure** Place the tips of
your middle fingers just below the
bridge of the nose. Press in lightly
close to the bone. Repeat in four
places, ending just below the nostrils.
You can press a little more firmly here
and hold for a little longer. Make sure
you keep to the sides of the nostrils
and do not obstruct your partner's
breathing. End by stroking the length
of the nose.

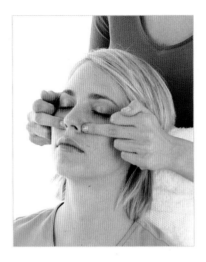

4 **squeezing** Massage the ears by
squeezing them between your fingers
and thumbs. Work from the tops of
the ears right round to the lobes, then
again along the inner line of the ear.
Return to the lobes and squeeze and
massage them thoroughly. End the
sequence by gently pulling at the
earlobes, then slide your fingers away.

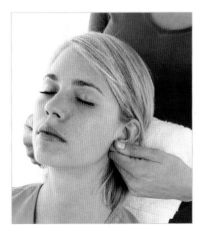

# The hair and scalp

These strokes should be performed with oil after the face sequence. Using oil feels luxurious and is good for the hair. If you choose not to use oil, these steps can follow on directly from the previous sequence on the head. In either case, the resting technique (Step 4) is the final contact for the whole massage.

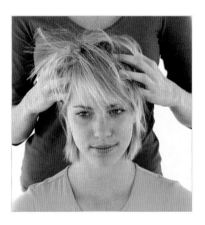

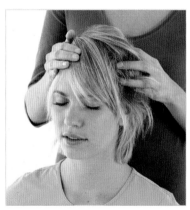

1 finger pressure If you are going to use oil, this is the time to apply it: pour some oil into your hands and apply it to your partner's hair, rubbing it in and massaging through to the ends. If you are not using oil, perform this sequence before working on the face. Begin shampooing movements over the scalp, applying pressure with the tips of your fingers for wonderful relaxation.

2 rotating Hold your partner's head with one hand, and place the tips of your fingers and thumb over the scalp. Spread your fingers and maintain that position. Rotate on the spot with your fingertips so that the scalp moves under your hand each time. Change hands so that you cover as much of the head as you can.

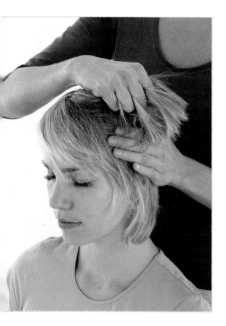

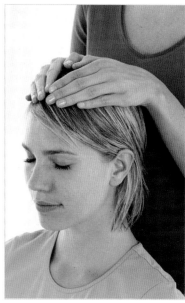

3  tugging Supporting the head with one hand, reach under the hair and grasp firmly at the roots. This prevents the technique from being painful. Tug fairly firmly without sliding, and work over the scalp tugging small handfuls of hair. This feels particularly good at the back of the head. Change hands to work over the remainder of the scalp.

4  resting To end, breathe calmly and place your hands just above the crown of your partner's head. Hold for a few moments, then gradually lower your hands so that they rest on top of the head. Breathe calmly once more, hold for a few moments, then slide your hands down over your partner's shoulders to end the massage.

# Indian head massage quick fix

If you only have a few moments in which to do Indian head massage, try the following sequence, which should ease tension in the neck and shoulders and stimulate the scalp. This can be done almost anywhere and provides a great energy boost.

1 **squeezing the shoulders** Stand behind your partner. Place your hands over the muscles along the tops of the shoulders. Lift and squeeze them between your fingers and thumbs. Grasp the muscles firmly to avoid pinching, lift and briefly hold. Work from the neck out toward the arms.

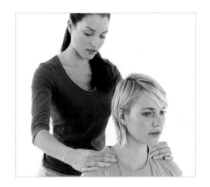

2 **percussion on the back** Form your hands into loose fists and pummel along the top of one shoulder toward the neck and back. Pummel lightly by the neck, then continue over the muscles down to the lower back. Repeat several times, then repeat on the other side of the spine. Keep your wrists relaxed in order to make the slightly dull, pummelling sound.

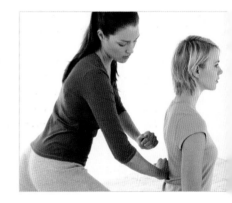

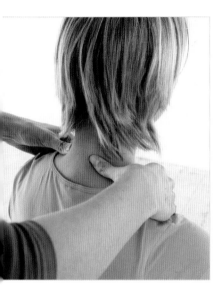

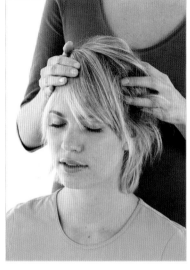

3 circling the neck Resting your fingers over the shoulders, place your thumbs at the base of the neck, about 1 in. (2.5 cm) away from the spine. Circle over the neck muscles up to the base of the skull. As you circle, the skin should also move under your thumbs. Repeat the movements several times to relax the neck.

4 rotating the scalp Supporting your partner's head with one hand, spread your other fingers wide and place the fingertips and thumb on the scalp. Rotate on the spot to create as much movement as you can. Fairly firm pressure is usually good. Move to different positions, then change hands to stimulate the remainder of the scalp.

# Self-massage

The following steps comprise Indian head-massage techniques to perform on yourself so that you can get the full benefits too. They are excellent when you feel stressed or headachy and are also very good to promote lustrous and healthy hair.

1 **rubbing the upper back** Reach over your shoulder with the opposite hand. Keeping your hand flat, rub vigorously across the top of the shoulder. The pressure should be fast, with enough friction to create warmth. Rub back and forth between the neck and arm, then repeat the movement over the other shoulder.

2 **percussion on the arms** Cup your hand around your upper arm, with your knuckles raised, making contact with the fingers and the heel of your hand. Cup quickly up and down the outer arm, working as far as the wrist to stimulate the circulation. Your movements should be quick, and keeping your wrist relaxed will produce the hollow cupping sound. Repeat over the other arm.

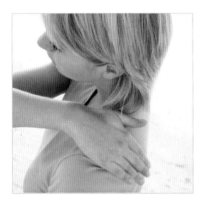

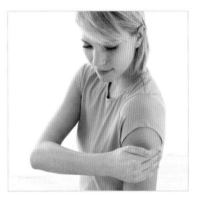

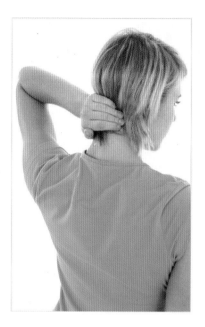

3 squeezing the neck Reach one hand behind your neck, with your fingers to one side of the spine and your heel to the other. Keep your knuckles raised over the spine itself. Starting at the base of the neck, squeeze and knead the muscles, working up to the base of the skull. Repeat with your other hand to even the pressure.

4 sawing the neck Using your index and middle fingers together, reach round to the base of the skull. Saw quickly and lightly over the muscles, working out toward the ear. Work backward and forward several times to relax the muscles, then repeat on the opposite side of the spine.

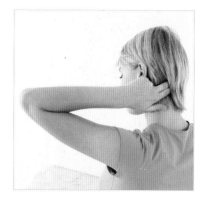

5 thumb pressure on the neck
Place your thumbs at the back of your head, with the fingers on the scalp for support. Your thumbs should be about 1 in. (2.5 cm) away from the spine and just under the base of the skull. Circle over the muscles with the balls of your thumbs, massaging toward the ears. This is great for reducing tension.

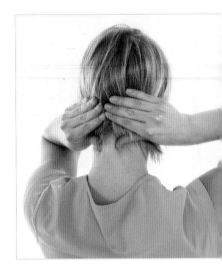

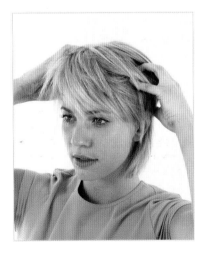

6 rotating over the head Place both hands over the scalp, knuckles raised, and fingers spread. Rotate on the spot while applying pressure, working over the scalp with both hands at once. This feels particularly good around the ears, temples and back of the head. Pressure should come from the balls of the fingers and thumbs.

**7 rubbing the head** Use the flat of your hand to rub vigorously over the scalp. Your movements should be sharp and brisk to stimulate the scalp and hair roots. Work over half the scalp with one hand, then change hands to cover the remainder of the head. Flick the ends of your hair as you rub so that it becomes quite ruffled.

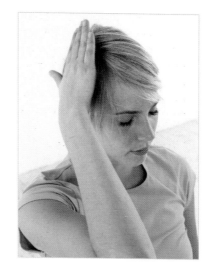

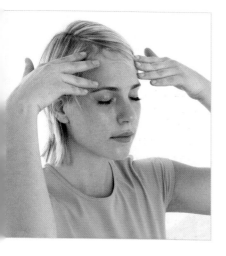

**8 finger pressure on the face** Place the tips of the fingers together in the middle of your forehead. Slowly draw your hands toward the temples, dragging your fingers slightly as you do so. This helps to relieve tension. Repeat in several lines across the forehead. It may help the relaxation process to keep your eyes closed.

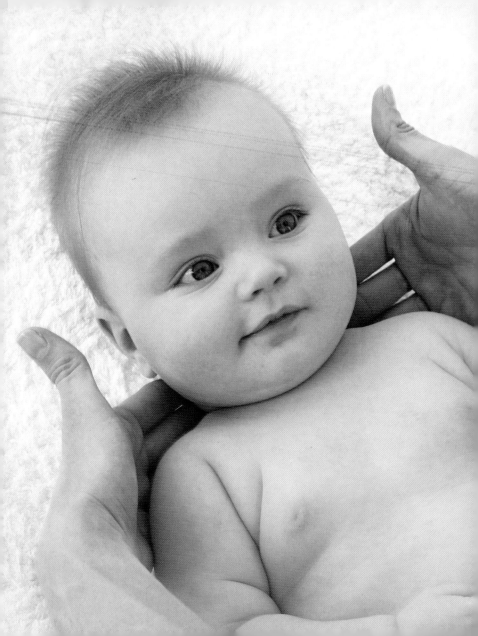

# Massage for special situations

When you massage, your partner might have particular needs (such as deep-tissue or sports massage), or you may wish to alter the focus of your techniques (say, to give massage to a pregnant woman or couple massage). On the following pages are some suggestions to incorporate into your massage or to be used on their own. If you use them on their own, remember to follow the principles of relaxing the muscles beforehand and using light strokes to close. Familiarize yourself with the techniques (see pages 48–101) before you begin, and ask your partner for feedback. That way you can build up your range and experience. Baby massage is presented as a self-contained full-body sequence for you and your baby to enjoy.

# Baby massage

Baby massage is a wonderful way of bonding with your baby. If you experienced massage through pregnancy, your baby will recognize the gentle rhythm of the movements. If not, massage is a great boost to the start of a baby's life. You can quite easily adapt techniques to suit your baby.

Babies thrive on touch. Massage stimulates their responses and increases the natural mother–baby connection.

*Baby massage just requires a mother's instinct and a little knowledge about the strokes and suitable oils.*

Your movements must be gentle and pleasurable, with lots of effleurage and very little pressure. While gentle stimulation of the muscles and joints is good for a baby's development, the movements need to be intuitive, your approach to massage flexible, and

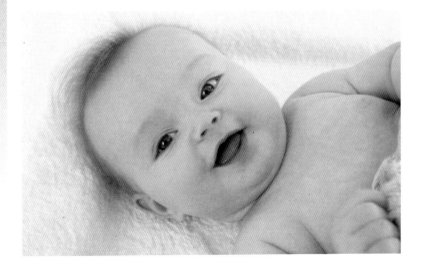

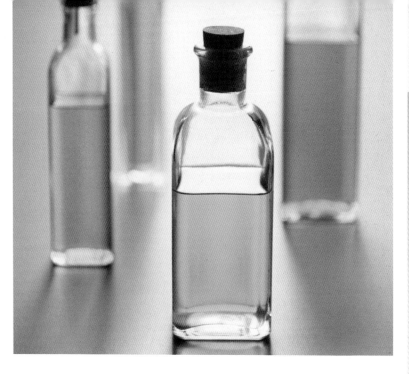

nothing should ever be forced—
especially if your baby does not feel like
keeping still. However, by developing a
relaxing routine, massage can help to
calm your baby. Massage only when
you feel calm yourself, and take time to
create a nurturing environment. Avoid
massage immediately after feeding.

## Suitable oils

A baby's skin is extremely sensitive, and
care should be taken with your choice

*Use only the purest of oils to moisturize
the skin which can be very delicate. For
essential oils, consult an aromatherapist.*

of oil: nothing strong-smelling or heavy,
and nothing that may cause sensitivity.
Use oils with a beneficial, moisturizing
effect. Sunflower oil mixed with a little
jojoba oil is perfect, or even some
calendula oil. Use organic oils wherever
possible. Essential oils should only be
used in a pre-blended mix.

# Application

Baby massage is beneficial to both mother and baby and is a special quiet time when you can bond. The strokes suggested in the massage sequence are for you to pick and choose from, as it is important not to tire or overstimulate your baby.

Make massage part of your daily routine from the outset, and continue for as long as your baby enjoys it. If you need guidance, it may help to attend baby massage classes. Oils should be kept simple, organic, and unfragranced (see page 279). Massage before rather than after a feed. Baby massage is about nurturing, touch, and increasing sensory stimulation, and should above all be playful, enjoyable, and fun.

Prepare everything you need beforehand, so have within reach oils (if you are using them), some tissues, wipes, diapers, and a blanket or towel. It often helps to build massage into your daily routine, for example before a bath, at bedtime, before a feeding, or nap. If you are using oil, do a patch test on the inside of your baby's elbow 24 hours beforehand to test for sensitivity, as a baby's skin is very delicate and may react. The massage can also be performed as a "dry massage" if you

## FOCUS POINTS

**Techniques:** The main strokes to use are gentle fingertip pressure, effleurage and light wringing.

**Movements:** These should be gentle, sensitive, soothing, and reassuring, with no heavy pressure and no fast or sudden strokes.

**Equipment:** You need somewhere comfortable where your back is supported; blankets, towels, and diapers, tissues and wipes at hand; soothing music to create a restful environment; pure vegetable oil.

**Feedback:** Your baby will give you instant feedback.

**Timing:** A baby massage should take 5–10 minutes, depending on your baby's age.

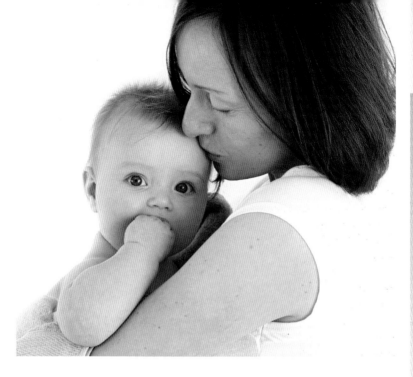

prefer, using less pressure to avoid any friction over the skin. It can even be done through clothes.

You can either sit on a chair with a back support or on the floor against the wall. The baby can either be on special padding on a table (but do bear safety in mind) or on a blanket on the floor in front of you. When your baby is very small, he or she is probably best on your knees or lap—it's a personal preference, but body contact is ideal.

*Make baby massage part of your daily routine. It should be loving and fun with as much body contact as possible.*

### CAUTION

Movements of the joints should not be attempted until after the first two months.

# Front of the body

Beginning on the front of the body is reassuring because you can keep eye contact with your baby which helps your baby to relax. Your strokes should be sweeping and flow one into another. Work intuitively and adapt or shorten the sequence as feels best.

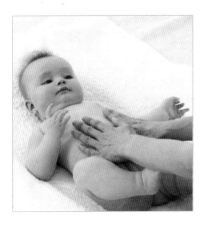

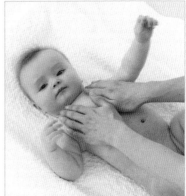

1 first contact Begin massage on the front so that you can maintain eye contact while your baby gets used to the movements. Find a position that works for you. Rub a little oil over your fingers, then position your hands on the abdomen, with your fingertips just below the navel. Pause for a few moments and simply observe.

2 effleurage Begin the massage with light sweeping strokes from the abdomen, up over the shoulders and down the ribcage to your starting position. Repeat several times to relax and reassure your baby. Mold your hands to the muscles and keep your movements gentle and rhythmic. Use very little pressure as you return on the downward stroke.

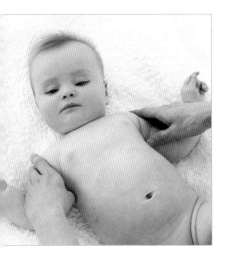

3 **effleurage** Repeat the effleurage strokes, this time sweeping up over the abdomen and continuing down the length of the arms. Squeeze the muscles very gently as part of the stroke. Repeat several times in different positions to spread the oil. Repeat in continuous, repetitive strokes.

4 **circling** As you complete the effleurage routine, continue over the hands and circle with your thumbs. Depending on your baby's position, you can either circle over the palms or the backs of the hands. The emphasis should be on relaxing the hand and opening out the fingers. Repeat several times.

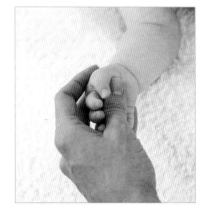

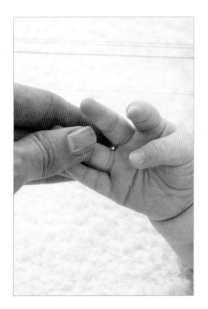

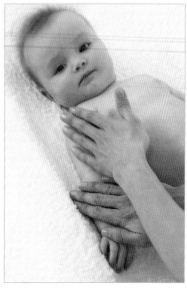

5  squeezing Gently squeeze each of your baby's fingers in turn, using the lightest of pressures to work down each finger to the tip. Either do this on both hands simultaneously or one at a time. "Bicycling" the fingers is another favorite. Gently move the wrists as well, so that the whole arm is involved in the strokes.

6  palm pressure Stroke with a little more pressure over each arm, using your hands alternately in a series of short sweeps. Begin at the wrist and massage right over the shoulder, cupping your hands around the joint. Pressure should come from the palms of the hands. Alternatively, use one hand for support and the other to massage upward over the arm.

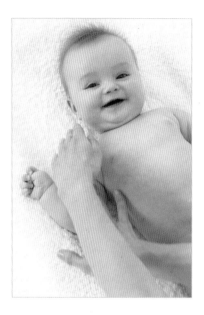

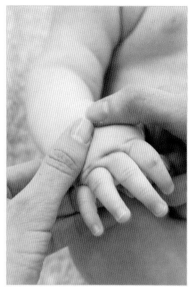

7 feathering Use your fingertips in a series of light feathering strokes down the arm. Work from shoulder to wrist. This is a light, playful stroke, but also serves to stimulate the skin and increase sensation. Keep your wrists raised and your hands relaxed so that the movement becomes like a series of waves.

8 circling Supporting the wrist from underneath, make little circles with your thumbs. Begin with both thumbs together in the center of the wrist, then circle outward in spirals over the joint. Pressure should be quite light with the balls of the thumbs, and your strokes should glide over the skin.

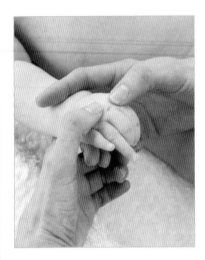

9 thumb circling Continue the circling strokes over the back of your baby's hand. Support it with your fingers underneath, and circle outward over the hands using the balls of your thumbs. The movements should be like spirals, with the strokes sliding over the skin. Repeat in several lines over the back of your baby's hand.

10 thumb circling Turn your baby's hand over, with the palm facing upward. Your fingers should support it from underneath. With the flats of your thumbs make small circles over the palm of the hand, so that you massage as much of the palm as possible. Your fingers underneath provide resistance. Squeeze the hand gently as you finish.

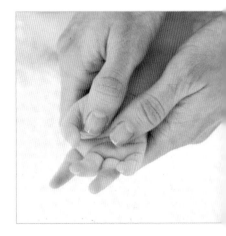

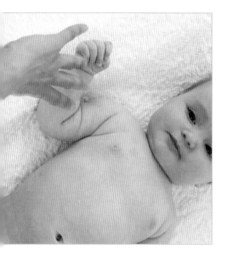

11 feathering Still supporting the hand, use light feathering strokes over the back of the hand and then turn it over. Continue feathering with your fingertips over the palm, and then feather the length of each finger in turn. The strokes will provide enjoyable sensations and skin stimulation for your baby. Then repeat all the movements on the other arm.

12 wringing Return to the chest, repeat the effleurage stroke, then wring lightly over the torso on the downward stroke. With the baby in a secure position, cross your hands to opposite sides of the ribs, with your hands molded around the chest. Slowly slide your hands toward each other and across to the other side. Repeat the movements to the lower abdomen.

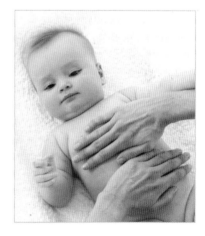

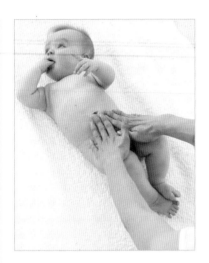

13 effleurage Use more oil if necessary, then effleurage outward over your baby's abdomen and this time down the legs. Squeeze gently to stimulate the muscles as part of the stroke, and wring and twist lightly over the skin. Repeat in several positions to spread the oil over as much of the skin as you can.

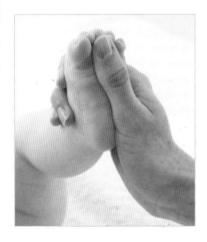

14 squeezing When you have completed the effleurage sequence, squeeze both feet between your hands, with your fingers on top and thumbs underneath. Massage the soles of the feet with your thumbs, or one foot at a time if this feels easier. Slide your hands, still gently squeezing, across the foot and over the toes.

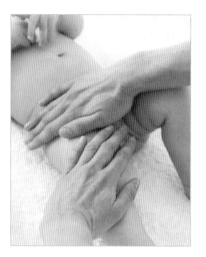

15 palm pressure With your palms flat, massage over one leg, beginning just above the ankle and ending over the hip. Then stroke, using slightly more pressure with the palms, in a series of short movements. Massage up the leg and over the hip, curving your hands around the joint. Repeat several more times to cover the whole thigh thoroughly.

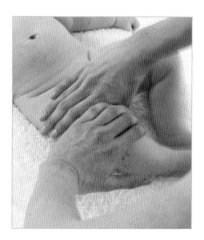

16 wringing Cup your hands around the outside of the thigh, with your fingers pointing inward. Gently slide both hands toward the center of the leg, and then cross to the opposite side. Wring lightly over the thigh, continuing down the leg as far as you can. You can apply a little pressure with this movement, as long as your hands glide rather than stick on the skin.

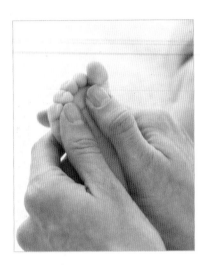

17 **thumb circling** Support your baby's foot in your hand, then make small circles over the sole with your thumbs. The circles should spiral under the foot. You can press gently at the base of the toes. Work over as much of the sole as you can, but do not apply pressure on the instep. If in doubt, simply massage the ball and over the heel.

18 **wringing** Place your thumbs underneath the foot, with your fingers over the top. Wring backward and forward over the foot, forming a complete movement with each hand. Continue to the toes and repeat several times, with your thumbs underneath providing resistance. This is good for relaxing the muscles.

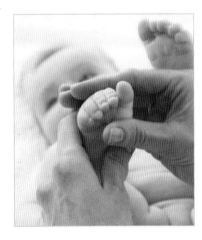

19 stretching Cup the heel in your hand and place your fingers against the sole of the foot. Gently press the foot downward but aim to stop before you feel resistance. Passive exercise is good for strengthening the joints. However, because a baby's joints can be very mobile, it is best to do this gently.

20 stretching Support the leg by holding it under the heel and at the knee. Gently push back toward the body to give a stretch at the hip. Do this several times. Your grip must be very light so you can relax before there is any resistance. Try again with the leg to the side. Lightly feather to the ankle and repeat on the other leg.

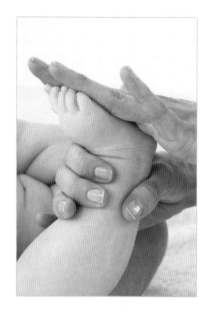

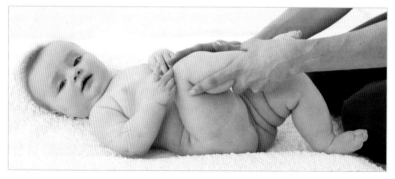

21 circling Return to the abdomen and effleurage as far as the baby's chest, then separate your hands and slide back down the sides of the ribs. From here make large circles over the ribs, sliding up the side of the body and circling back down again. Repeat several times with your fingers splayed wide and your hands relaxed, sliding over the skin.

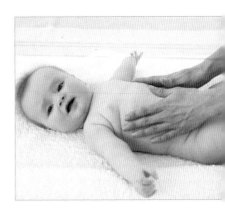

22 effleurage Place your thumbs together in the center of the chest, just beneath the collarbone. Apply a little more oil, if you need to. Slowly stroke out over the top of the chest to the shoulders with the balls of your thumbs. Round your hands over the shoulders and repeat several times.

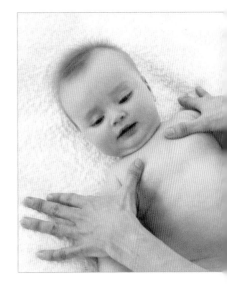

23 finger pressure Reach around the back of your baby's neck with your fingertips, index fingers cradling the baby's skull. Place your middle and fourth fingers on the muscles to the sides of the spine. Very, very gently, press the muscles with your fingertips and massage upward to the base of the skull.

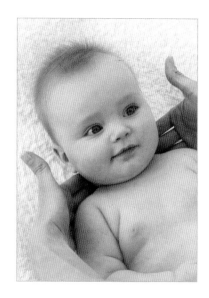

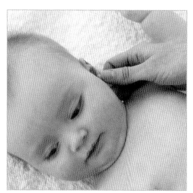

24 squeezing With your hands still cradling the head, stroke the cheeks with your thumbs in a circular motion back toward the ears. Then gently squeeze the earlobes between your thumbs and index fingers, and stroke around and behind the ears. These are intended to be small, pleasurable, and reassuring movements.

# The face

Massage over the baby's face and scalp should be extremely light, avoiding
any oil near the eyes. Make it playful so that the whole massage experience
is enjoyable and something you both look forward to. This is a time for
sharing eye contact, encouraging noises, and smiles.

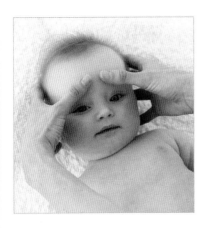

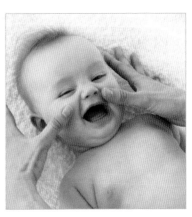

1 effleurage With the baby's head
supported once more, very gently
stroke over the forehead with the
balls of your thumbs. Start with your
thumbs together in the center of the
forehead and then slowly draw them
apart. Repeat several times, keeping
your movements well away from the
eyes. You may need to use a little more
oil so your thumbs glide over the skin.

2 effleurage Place your thumbs over
the cheeks and repeat the effleurage
strokes, working over the cheekbones
toward the ears. Your thumbs should
glide smoothly over the skin. Give the
apples of the cheeks a little pinch to
keep your baby smiling. Repeat in
several lines over the face.

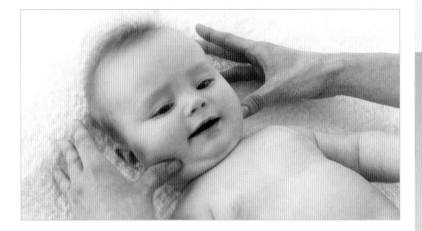

3 **effleurage** Move your thumbs to the chin, crooking your index fingers underneath and placing the balls of your thumbs in the center. Slowly draw your hands out along the line of the jaw. Repeat several times and, on the last stroke, give the earlobes a few gentle squeezes.

4 **effleurage** Place both palms just above the hairline, with your fingers facing the center of the head. Gently stroke over your baby's hair toward the back of the head. Use your hands alternately for a soft, relaxing rhythm. This is a great time for lots of eye contact and soothing sounds.

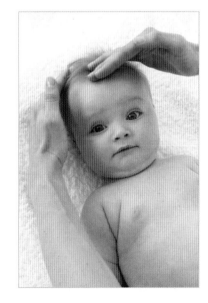

# Back of the body

Once relaxed, your baby should be happy to have massage on the back.
Make sure the body is fully supported. Keep your strokes sweeping, short,
and light, with one flowing into another, and shorten the sequence if you
or your baby tires. Adapt the strokes to suit your baby's position.

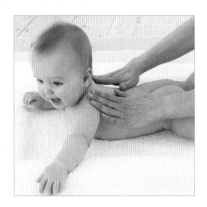

1 effleurage Find a comfortable
position for massage so that your
baby is supported. Rub a little oil over
your fingers and effleurage over the
back. Begin with your fingers together
by the lower back, glide up over the
shoulders, then back down the sides
of the body. The strokes should be
soothing, with your hands molded to
the shape of the muscles.

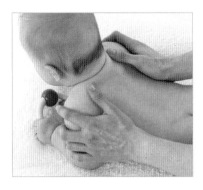

2 circling Repeat the effleurage stroke
and, as your hands divide, circle out
across the shoulders with your thumbs.
The circles should be continuous
spirals, with your thumbs gliding over
the skin. Repeat the circling movements
several times. Start 1 in. (2.5 cm) out
from the spine and massage toward
the arms.

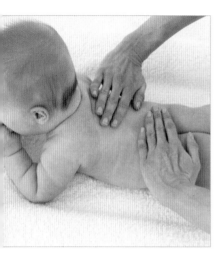

3 wringing Place your hands just under the armpits on opposite sides of the ribs. Slowly draw them toward each other so that they cross to the other side. Lightly wring down to the lower back. Your touch should be light and your movements should slide over the skin without pulling. Repeat over the back several times.

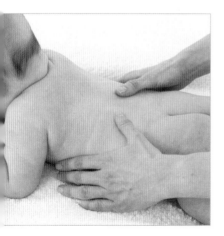

4 circling As you return to the lower back, circle out over the top of the buttocks using large, broad circles with your thumbs. Begin 1 in. (2.5 cm) away from the spine and spiral across the skin. By using the sides of your thumbs you can ensure that the pressure remains even and does not dig in. Repeat several times.

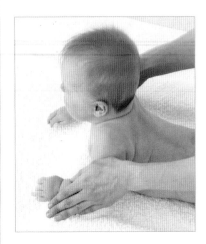

5 **effleurage** Apply a little more oil to your hands and effleurage over the baby's back once more, this time sweeping down the backs of the arms to the hands. Slide over the hands and the fingers in one broad, continuous movement. Repeat several times to sufficiently oil and stimulate the skin.

6 **rocking** Place your hands around the upper arm. Gently rock the muscles between your hands, working down to the wrist. Keep your hands molded to the muscles, and relax your movements at the elbow. Adjust your hands to accommodate your baby's position, and simply rock as much of the arm as you can.

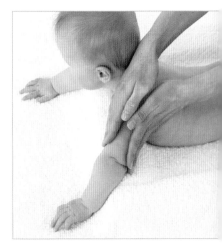

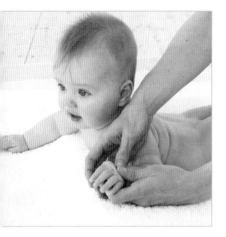

7 thumb-rolling Support your baby's hand, then roll your thumbs over the back of the hand toward the fingers, spreading them wide as you do so. Thumb-roll in several lines, using the sides of the thumbs for softer movements. Circle very gently between the tendons and around the knuckles.

8 squeezing Squeeze the fingers gently between your index finger and thumb. Massage each one in turn, working down the finger and over the tip. You can also rub and roll the fingers between your own. Feather down the arm from shoulder to fingertips, then repeat all the movements over the other arm.

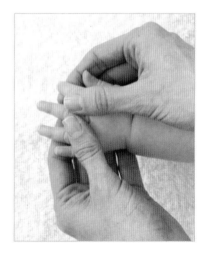

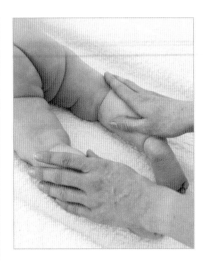

9 effleurage Rub a little oil over your fingers if you need to, and place your fingertips together at your baby's lower back. Glide upward with your fingers together, then separate your hands to sweep over the buttocks and down the legs. Repeat the strokes several times, working right down to and over the feet.

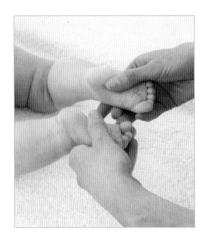

10 squeezing After your last effleurage stroke, squeeze over the soles of the feet, with your fingers supporting them underneath and your thumbs on the sole. Gently squeeze the feet between your fingers and thumbs, and especially squeeze over the fleshy part of the soles. Remember to avoid the insteps.

11 **wringing** Place your hands on either side of the thigh, fingers facing inward. Slowly slide your hands past each other to reach the opposite side of the leg. Continue wringing up and down the thigh as far as the knee. Keep your wrists relaxed and your hands molded around the muscles.

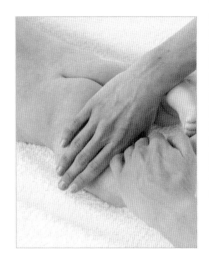

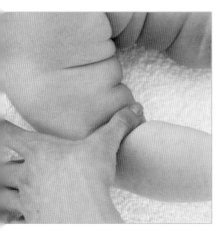

12 **thumb pressure** To massage over the back of the knee, change your strokes to movements with your thumbs. Support the knee from underneath if necessary and smooth outward over the crease with the sides of your thumbs. Curl your thumbs around the sides of the knee before repeating the strokes. Then continue wringing down the calf to the ankle.

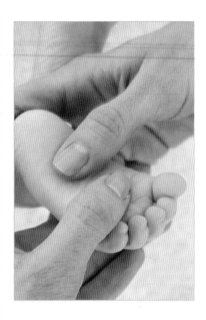

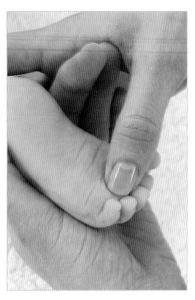

13 **wringing** Cradle the baby's foot in your hands, with your fingers underneath and your thumbs over the sole. Wring backward and forward across the foot with both hands at the same time. Then slide to the center and back again. Your movements should glide over the skin while your fingers remain molded around the foot.

14 **thumb pressure** Still supporting the foot in your hands, gently circle and press under the base of the toes. Use the tip of your thumb to press lightly between and around the joints and to circle over the pads of the toes. This is a nice movement to relax the feet. Remember to keep the pressure gentle and soothing.

15 pulling Cradle the foot in one hand and gently pull each toe in turn. Wiggle down from the base of each toe to the tip. Give little presses and squeezes between your fingers and thumb to make the movements fun. Squeeze and hold the ball of each toe before sliding over the tip.

16 feathering Supporting the leg with one hand, feather along its length with the other hand in light movements to stimulate the skin. Short strokes with the tips of the fingers feel best, and are relaxing and reassuring. Repeat several times over the foot. Then repeat all the movements on the other leg.

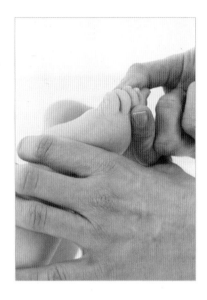

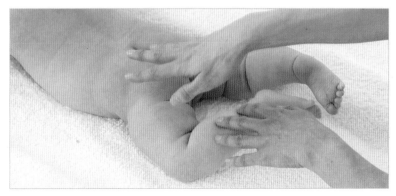

17 plucking This is a slight variation on the plucking stroke. Support your baby under the shoulder. Place your thumb and index finger at the back of the neck, on the muscles to either side of the spine. Gently raise your hand and slide your fingers over the skin as you "pluck" into the air. This must be very gentle, without squeezing or pinching. Repeat twice more to relax the neck.

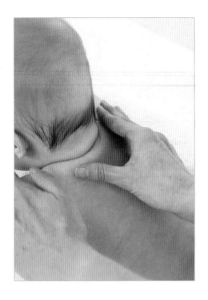

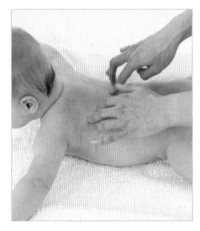

18 percussion Gently tap with the balls of your fingers, using small, light movements like raindrops, the length of the back. Avoid tapping over the spine itself. Work from the shoulders down to the lower back in a series of playful movements. Repeat several times.

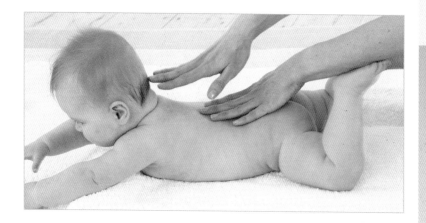

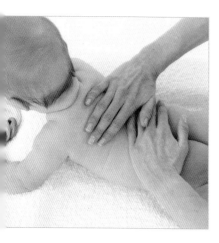

19 **feathering** Lightly feather down the spine with your fingertips, working from the shoulders to the lower back. Keep your wrists relaxed in a series of flowing strokes, using your hands alternately. These movements should be calming, relaxing and nurturing.

20 **resting** To end the massage, rest your hands lightly on the back and pause for a few moments. One hand should be between the shoulder blades and the other over the sacrum, the bony triangle at the base of the spine. Breathe calmly for a few moments and focus on the contact between your hands and your baby's skin. Then turn the baby back over to face you.

# Couple massage

Massage can be a lot of fun. It is great for helping couples to de-stress and get physically and emotionally closer. The basic techniques remain, but adding sensual movements and nuances can turn a massage into a romantic dance. Sensual strokes are playful, light, lingering, and come from the heart.

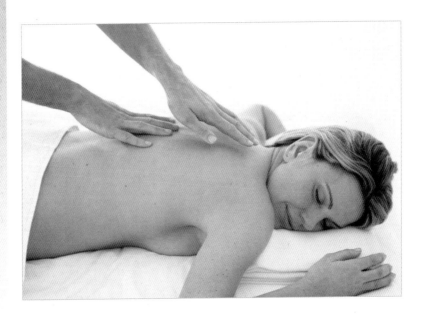

1 feathering the skin Feathering—a connecting stroke—can become a caress. We often take our partners for granted, so here is a chance to rediscover their skin. Use your fingers, fingertips, and nails to stroke gently over your partner's body. The lighter the touch, the more it stimulates the skin. Take time to explore the outline of muscles and joints in an affirming, caring way.

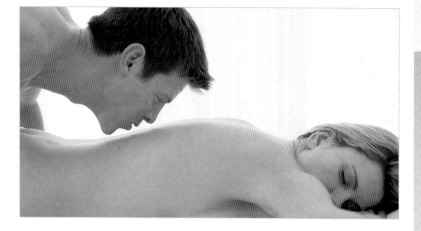

2 **blowing on the skin** This is a
romantic touch for the end of any
sequence. After massaging the muscles
gently, blow over the surface of the
skin. The closer you are to the body, the
warmer your breath will be. This is great
as a relaxing technique or to stimulate
your partner's skin. Try it over the
limbs, back, or nape of the neck.

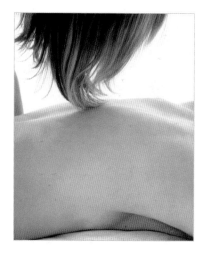

3 **flicking the hair** Use this at the
end of any massage sequence. The
longer your hair, the easier it is, but
you can still be inventive. Use the ends
to brush and flick over your partner's
skin. This feels great over broad areas
like the back. Long brushing strokes
work best.

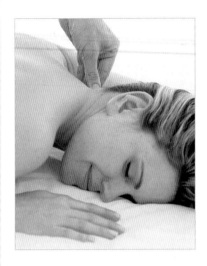

4 kneading the neck Be creative with your massage. Use closeness and intimacy to massage at unexpected moments, as a way of expressing tenderness and appreciation. It is hard to feel loving when you are tense. Knead the nape of your partner's neck between fingers and thumb—as always, avoiding any direct movements over the spine.

5 finger pressure on the face Massaging the face feels fantastic, but adding soft, caressing strokes makes it special. Use the balls and tips of your fingers to draw softly across the features of your partner's face. Work outward from the center with slow, languid strokes. Take time to trace around the eyes, nose, and mouth. Trace softly over the eyelids and lips.

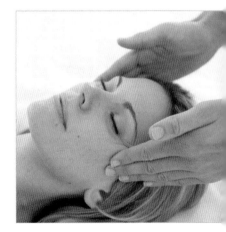

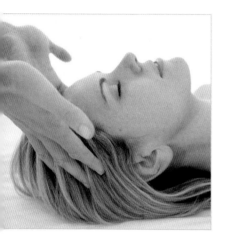

6 **pulling the hair** Massaging the scalp feels great, and so does tugging gently at the hair roots. Make the strokes playful. Stroke from the roots to the very tips, threading the hair between your fingers. Curl the ends, pull very gently and ruffle your partner's hair.

7 effleurage on the back
Be inventive with techniques that you already know. Try different ways of effleuraging over the back, varying your pressure, position and tempo. Hands and fingertips are familiar, so why not try the forearms or feet? Keep full contact with the muscle contours for the best results.

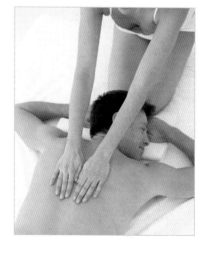

# Pregnancy massage

Massage is great during pregnancy. It helps to relieve backache, neck tension, swollen ankles, tired legs, and painful breasts, and you can contribute to your partner's well-being. At the same time the baby will start to respond to the familiar sensations and routines.

**CAUTION**

Pressure needs to be much lighter during pregnancy to avoid overstimulation. Avoid putting pressure over the lower back or abdomen during the first four months.

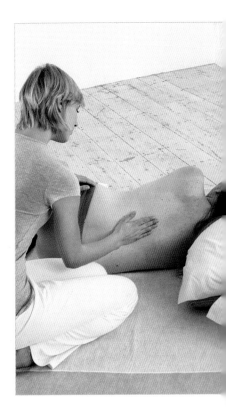

1  circling the lower back The lower back can get very uncomfortable during pregnancy. Try this while your partner lies on her side, supporting her with pillows for comfort. Place one hand on the body for support and the other hand flat in the hollow of the back. Circle slowly counterclockwise so that your hand slides over the skin, using a little oil to help. Use broad, relaxing strokes, but avoid any firm or uneven pressure.

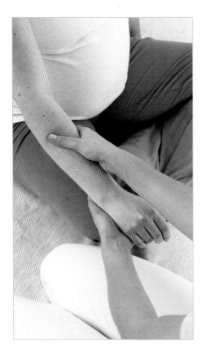 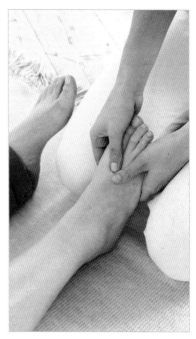

2 squeezing the arms Rub some oil over your hands. With your partner supported, you can then squeeze over the arm. Squeeze with both hands cupped around the forearm. Release the pressure at the elbow and continue toward the shoulder. Repeat the strokes slowly so that they feel nicely soothing. Repeat on the other side.

3 thumb pressure on the feet
The feet are another part of the body that get really tired, especially toward the end of the pregnancy. With the legs resting, you can massage over the feet, circling around the joints and squeezing between the tendons. Use your thumbs to circle the ankles as well. Apply a little pressure over the ball of the foot, but avoid overstimulation.

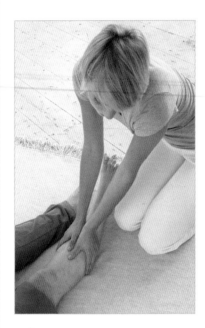

4 squeezing the legs With your
partner's legs resting, apply some oil
to your hands and squeeze up over the
calf muscles, circle around the knee
and continue squeezing up over the
thigh. This helps to relieve tiredness
in the legs. You might need to change
your position when working over the
thigh. If your partner has varicose
veins, simply brush lightly over the
skin instead.

5 finger pressure on the back
With your partner on her side and
supported, use your fingers to slide
away from the muscles at the side of
the spine. Splay your fingers and slide
between the ribs, sliding over the
muscles in a raking movement. Your
partner will need to turn over so you
can repeat this on the other side.

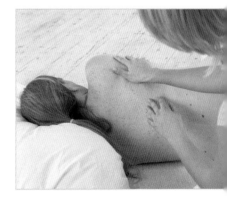

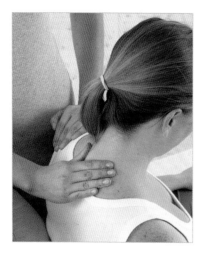

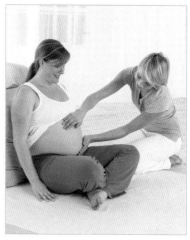

6 kneading the neck With your partner supported in a comfortable position, you can knead the neck muscles with one hand and keep body contact with the other. Knead on either side of the spine with your thumb and fingers, keeping your knuckles raised to avoid the spine itself. Kneading slowly is best; there should be no heavy pressure around this area.

7 effleurage on the abdomen You may be doing this massage already. If not, try spreading some oil over your fingers and make big, slow clockwise circles over the abdomen. Use the flats of your hands and mould them to your partner's belly. Over time you will be able to see or feel the baby respond.

**CAUTION**

Only attempt this massage step after the first four months of pregnancy.

# Deep-tissue massage

This involves specialized techniques over muscle and connective tissue. While the increased pressure can be deeply satisfying, you need to apply caution when using it. The techniques can release deep-seated tension and address postural problems. The suggestions below give a flavor of this massage style.

1 **elbow pressure on the back**
Apply oil over your partner's back. Supporting the body, lean over and place a rounded elbow on the muscles on the opposite side of the spine. Apply pressure upward over the muscles as far as the upper back, and round the movement over the shoulder using your forearm. Avoid too sharp an angle at the elbow, so that the pressure feels firm rather than digging in.

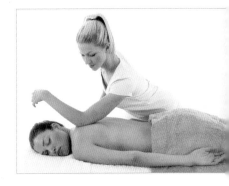

2 **finger pressure on the shoulders** Use a double finger press to work around your partner's shoulder blade. Begin with one hand over the top of the shoulder, and place your other hand on top to increase the pressure. Slide your hands right around the outline of the shoulder blade as you press to relax the muscles and stimulate the circulation.

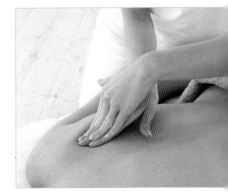

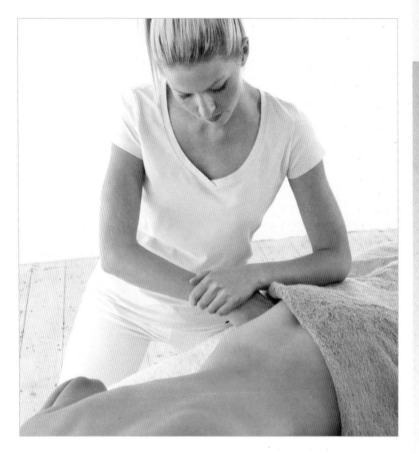

3 knuckle pressure on the
   buttocks Use both hands to work
   into fleshy muscular areas, such as the
   buttocks. Form your hand into a fist
   and press with your knuckles, placing
   your other hand on top to increase
   the pressure. Lean in with your body
   weight and circle, knead and press over
   the muscles. Take great care not to
   exert pressure over bony areas.

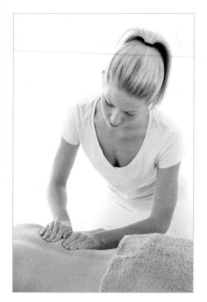

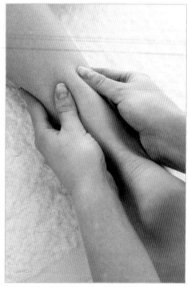

4 finger pressure on the back

Place the fingertips of both hands over the muscles to the side of the spine. Press down into the muscles, at the same time rolling your fingers over the muscle bands. This is done as a slow, deep movement, avoiding pressure over the spine itself. The stroke works best where there is increased muscle tone.

5 thumb-rolling the calves

Support the leg at the ankle and place your thumbs just above the ankle bone and to either side of the tendons. Roll up toward the calf muscles, applying pressure with the balls of your thumbs. Repeat in several movements, applying firm, but not painful pressure. Press just behind and close into the bone for the best results.

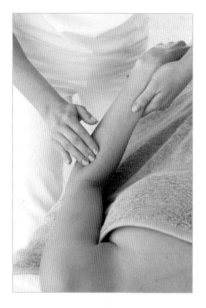

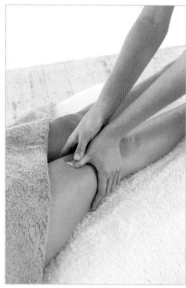

6 vibration over the forearms

Locate the muscular area between the bones of the forearm. Place the balls of your fingers over the muscles, press down and vibrate on the spot. This increases the penetration of any pressure, so it must only be done over fleshy muscles. Movements last for a few moments before you release them. Work over the forearm then repeat the movements on the other side.

7 thumb pressure on the thighs

Place your thumb on the thigh, roughly 2 in. (5 cm) above the kneecap. Slide over the crest of the muscles and, using the ball of your thumb, apply pressure in the direction of the hip. The movement should follow the line of the muscles and end at least 2 in. (5 cm) below the hip. Always start with light pressure, and check any increase with your partner. Repeat on the other leg.

# Sports massage

Many athletes use sports massage to keep fit. It helps prevent injury through muscle relaxation and passive exercise of the joints and is also excellent after sport to help rid the body of excess lactic-acid. It is specialized, but the following movements will give you some basic techniques.

1 rotating the hips Bend your partner's leg back toward the body by lifting it below the ankle and the knee. Press against the lower leg and bring the knee toward the chest until you feel resistance. At this point, rotate the leg at the hip so that you provide a stretch. Explore your partner's range of movement and repeat, gradually increasing the range of the rotations.

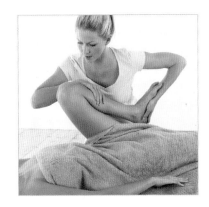

2 finger pressure on the knees Press around the kneecap with the balls of your fingers, working around its outline by pressing and circling on the spot. Your other hand should provide guidance and resistance. Ensure that you do not work over the kneecap itself. This is a good technique for increasing stimulation of the joint, but it is not suitable where there are any known knee problems.

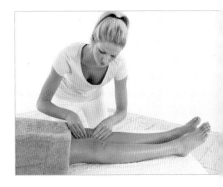

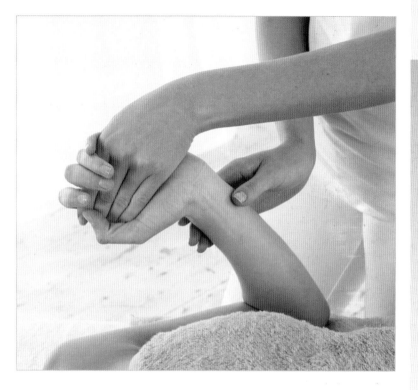

3 rotating the wrists Support your
partner's arm at the elbow. Grasp the
hand securely and use your palm to
apply pressure. This is good for passive
exercise of the joint. You can then
slowly rotate the hand at the wrist in
both directions, while applying pressure
to increase the mobility of the joint.

4 squeezing the legs Calf muscles can get very tight, so you can help to increase the circulation by adapting the familiar squeezing technique. Your partner should rest their ankle over your shoulder, giving you freedom to use both hands. Squeeze over the calf muscles toward the back of the knee, using full hand contact. Simply be careful not to exert undue pressure on the knee.

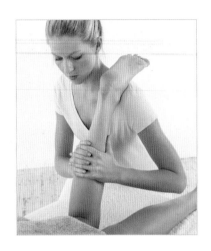

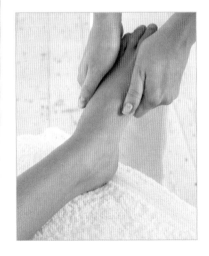

5 squeezing the feet Place both hands on either side of the foot. Squeeze tightly between the fingers and the heels of your hands. Then stretch the tendons by pulling down on one side of the foot, while pushing upward on the other side. Try to get as much movement as you can, then reverse the direction of your hands. Repeat until the muscles relax and become more pliable.

6 palm pressure on the shoulders Bend your partner's arm behind the back to expose the shoulder blade. Support under the shoulder with one hand, then spread your thumb and index finger and slide your other hand as far under the blade as feels comfortable. Apply pressure with the palm of your hand and the web between your index finger and thumb. This is great for relaxing the shoulder.

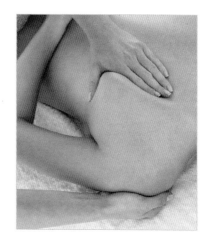

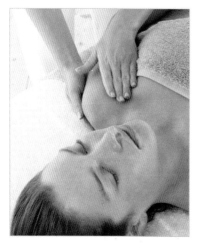

7 rubbing the shoulders Place both hands over the ball of the shoulder, one on top and the other underneath. Rub vigorously between your hands to increase the circulation. Rub around the joint and over the upper arm in a series of brisk movements. Contact should be with the palms of the hands. This is very good as a warm-up before physical activity.

# Beauty massage

The aesthetic benefits of massage are numerous. Relaxed muscles freed from metabolic waste improve the appearance of the face, while increased circulation and the use of nourishing oils make the skin glow. Feeling good in turn makes you look good, producing that priceless glow from within.

1 circling the temples Place the tips of your fingers over both your partner's temples. Apply a little pressure and circle back toward you, so that you lift the features and stretch the skin. It is important always to stroke so that you lift *away* from the face and encourage the features to appear more relaxed and open. Work in half-circles so that you avoid any pressure *toward* the face.

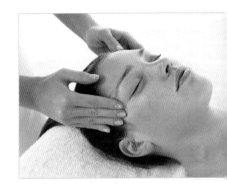

2 squeezing the eyebrows Place your thumbs and index fingers on the ridge of the eyebrows. Working from the inner line of the brows, lift and pinch at regular intervals out toward the temples. This increases circulation to the muscles, but also helps to relax the forehead and eyes. Repeat several times over the browline, keeping your fingers steady. Remember to work well away from the eyes.

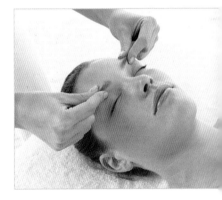

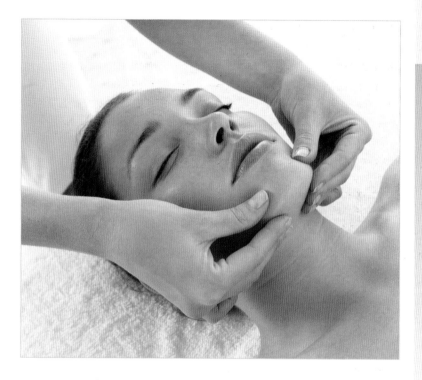

3 squeezing the jaw This helps to increase jaw definition. Apply a little oil to your fingers, if necessary, and place your fingertips under the jawline, with your thumbs together in the center of the chin. Squeeze the jawbone as you slide your hands outward along the line of the jaw. As you do so, you gently stretch the skin and stimulate the muscles.

4 circling the jaw Place your fingertips over the muscles at the angle of your partner's jaw. These muscles are very often tense and give the face a rather cross, determined look. Apply pressure with the balls of your fingers and stroke in big, broad circles over the muscles, while encouraging your partner to relax the jaw. Press with your fingertips wherever you feel any particularly tight spots.

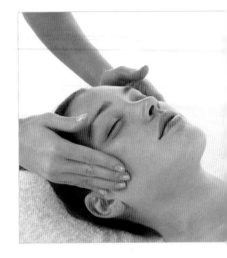

5 effleurage on the eyelids With your partner's eyes closed, place the balls of your middle fingers very lightly over the eyelids, close to the bridge of the nose. Steadily and gently draw your fingers over the lids, taking care not to press down on the eyes. Make sure that you have enough oil on your fingertips not to drag the skin—but not so much that you irritate the eyes.

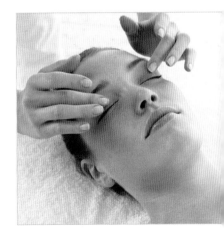

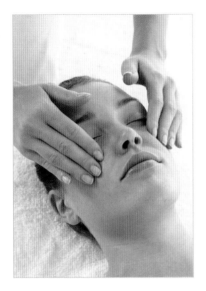

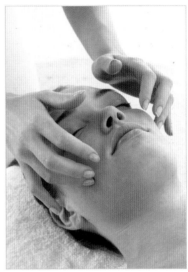

6 circling the cheeks Place the balls of your fingers over the cheeks. Massage in small, spiralling circles over the cheeks from the nose toward the ears. This should stimulate the muscles and improve the circulation without dragging the skin. Repeat in three horizontal lines, always ending on a positive, upward stroke.

7 percussion on the cheeks and jaw Lightly tap over the cheeks and jaw like drops of falling rain. Use the balls of your fingers to keep the movements soft. Keep your hands steady, with your wrists raised. Your movements should be rapid and light. This stimulates the skin, improves the circulation, and imparts a beautiful, healthy glow.

# Energy-field massage

All massage treating the whole person is healing. A holistic approach takes into account the body, mind, emotions, and spiritual dimensions of each person. Working on one particular aspect can affect the balance of the whole, and healing is all about achieving balance.

## Energy centers and fields

As we have seen *chakras* are communication points of energy (see pages 246–247). Each of the seven major energy centers is believed to have a particular location, is associated with certain physical aspects and has a different color and sound vibration. In addition, there are various energy fields surrounding each individual, known as auras. Some people can see or read auras and the colors within them. The energy field closest to the body is known as the etheric body, and you may be able to feel this by holding your hand about 6–9 in. (15–23 cm) above the skin. It is believed that energy imbalances affect our physical well-being and may even be a cause of illness. Balancing energy can help us regain health, and there are some healers who work solely on energy fields. By developing a healing touch you can enhance your massage.

Energy-field techniques work both on and above the body. Developing sensitivity is the first step, as well as empathy with and respect for your massage partner. Empty your mind, focus on your hands and note any sensations that you feel. Be objective and simply observe. Try the following techniques after massaging the muscles, or beforehand, to help your partner relax. With practice you will gain confidence and be able to refine your technique.

# The aura

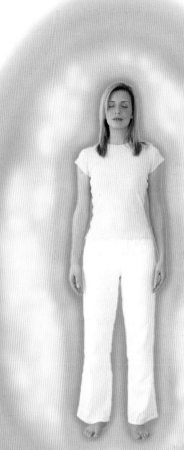

**The energy fields** that surround the body are collectively known as the aura.

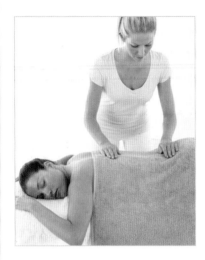

1 resting on the back After massaging the back, end the sequence by placing one hand between your partner's shoulder blades and the other over the sacrum, the bony triangle at the base of the spine. Breathe calmly, empty your mind and focus on the sensations in your hands. Imagine positive energy flowing out through your palms. This feels comforting and helps to connect upper and lower back.

2 energy-sensing on the back Place your hand flat on your partner's sacrum. Slowly raise your hand about 4–6 in. (10–15 cm) above the body. Circle counterclockwise above the sacrum and note any sensations in your palm. Gradually lower your hand so that it rests over the sacrum again. This relaxes the lower back.

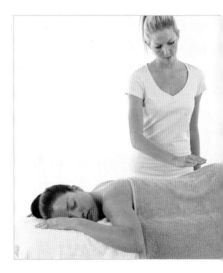

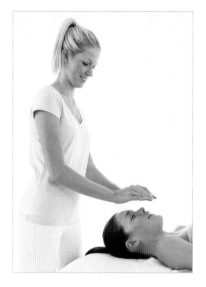

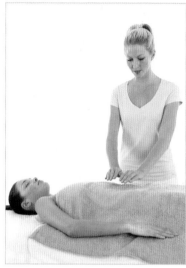

3 resting the eyes This is good after massaging the face and feels deeply relaxing. Cup your hands and place them about 6 in. (15 cm) above the eyes, shading them from the light. Breathe calmly and imagine positive energy flowing through your palms. Keep your hands steady and your mind still. Your partner may notice the warmth from your hands.

4 resting over the abdomen Try this after massaging the abdomen. It is particularly good if your partner is experiencing any sensitivity, and is a very centering technique. Hold your hands just above the abdomen. Note any sensations that you pick up. Gradually lower your hands so that they rest flat on either side of the navel. Breathe out positive energy through your palms.

5 resting at the head This is good for headaches or mental tension. Rest your hands on either side of your partner's head, with your palms facing inward. Let them simply relax. Note any sensations that you feel and imagine positive energy flowing out through your palms. Move your hands slightly further away from the head and repeat, gradually getting further away each time.

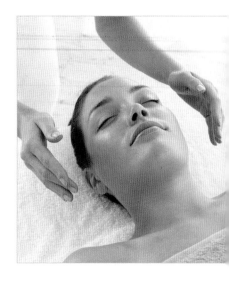

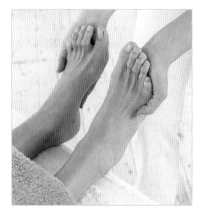

6 resting at the feet This helps to center or ground your partner after a massage by drawing attention down to the feet. After you have massaged them, place your hands in a relaxed position over the soles. Relax the palms of your hands and feel the contact with your partner's feet. Focus your attention simply on the points of contact between you.

7 energy-sensing over the head
Stand behind your partner. Place your hands together roughly 12 in. (30 cm) above the crown of the head. Relax your palms and note any sensations that you feel. Gradually lower both hands so that they cup the crown. Note the change in sensation as you get closer to the body. Imagine positive energy flowing through your hands.

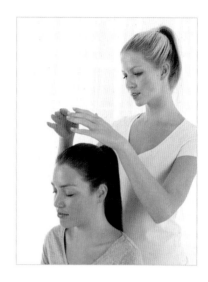

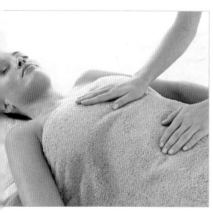

8 resting over the front of the body Place one hand flat against the chest and the other over the abdomen. Simply rest. Note the rise and fall of the breath, and keep your own breathing calm and steady. Note any changes to your partner's breathing and concentrate on the warmth of your hands. This is very helpful and balancing if your partner is emotionally upset.

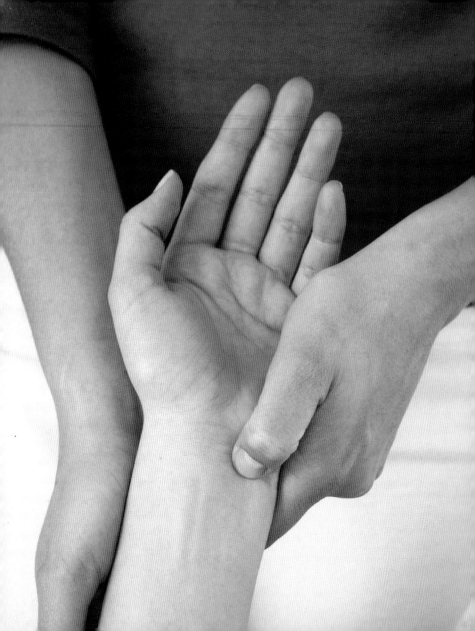

# Common ailments

Massage has been used as a home remedy for years. On the following pages are some common ailments and suggestions for massage techniques to help them. At the very least, massage provides comfort from pain, and the reduction in stress often helps alleviate symptoms. The most useful techniques have been included, regardless of their tradition. In the case of acupressure points and meridians, you can choose whether a Chinese massage (see pages 156–199) or clothed shiatsu (see pages 200–243) approach is more convenient. These suggestions are not a substitute for medical help, particularly important in ailments affecting a baby or young child.

# Tension headaches

Headaches are very common and can be caused by eyestrain, posture, diet, and stress. Massage can be extremely beneficial for tension headaches. However, they can have more serious causes, and medical attention should always be sought for prolonged or serious headaches.

rotating over the scalp To relieve the feeling of tightness, place your hand in position over your partner's scalp. Contact should be made with the balls of the fingers and thumbs. Circle on the spot and get as much movement of the scalp as possible. Repeat in several positions to increase the circulation, using your other hand to provide support. Start lightly and increase your pressure as the tension eases.

finger pressure on the eye sockets Locate GB 1, which is roughly one finger-width out from the eye sockets. Find the small depressions in the bone and circle gently with the tips of your middle fingers. Any pressure should be back toward the hairline, away from the face. Slowly press into the points, hold for a few moments and release. Continue circling until the tension eases. This is a favorite shiatsu remedy.

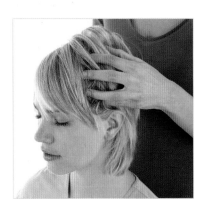

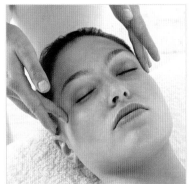

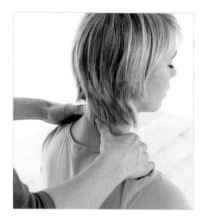

## thumb pressure on the neck

Lying face down can be uncomfortable with a headache, so try relieving neck tension—the cause of many headaches—with your partner sitting up. Place your thumbs over the muscles on either side of the spine and circle up toward the base of the skull. Press under the skull, massaging tense spots, and work out toward the ears.

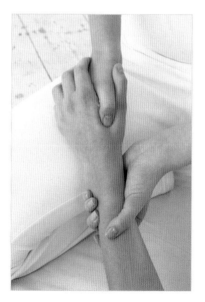

## thumb pressure on the hands

This spot can relieve headaches, especially if they have digestive origins. Place your thumb over the web between your partner's index finger and thumb, with your middle finger underneath. Locate the small depression signifying LI 4. Press and circle over the spot with the tip of your thumb, applying resistance with your finger. Check the pressure and repeat on the other hand.

### CAUTION

Do not use point LI 4 during pregnancy.

# Blocked sinus

A blocked sinus can range from feeling slightly stuffy to very intense pain. Pressure points work best to try and ease the congestion. Begin gently until you see some results. You may need to repeat the movements over several days for your partner to feel relief.

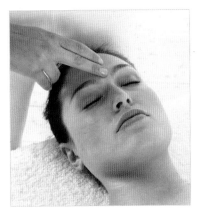

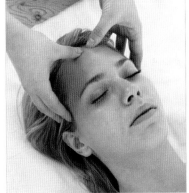

finger pressure between the brows Place the tip of your middle finger over the Yintang point, which is located between your partner's brows. Position your finger, press gently, hold, and then release. Repeat several times, pressing and releasing slowly and evenly until some relief is felt. This also helps to calm the system.

thumb pressure on the head Work up the bladder meridian in a line from the eyebrows to the hairline and over the back of the head. Press with the flats of both thumbs in a steady rhythm: position, press, hold, release. This helps to clear the sinuses. To relieve discomfort, press in several vertical lines working upward over the forehead.

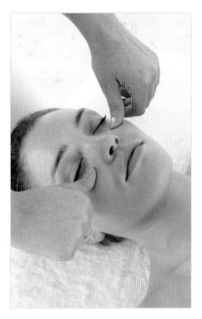

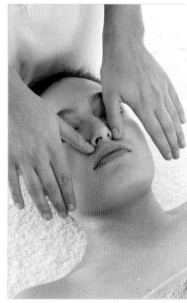

**thumb pressure on the eye sockets** Press along the lower eye-socket ridge using the sides of your thumbs at even intervals. About one-third of the way along you will feel a slight depression in the bone. This is the location of St 1. Press in and hold for a few moments to clear the sinuses. Continue working out steadily toward the temples.

**thumb pressure by the nostrils** Press Co 20, which lies in the depression on either side of the nostrils. Use the balls of your thumbs to press downward and slightly in toward the nostrils. This offers good sinus relief, although make sure your pressure does not restrict your partner's breathing. Press and hold for a few moments, then release.

# Dark circles

Dark circles under the eyes can be due to lack of exercise, poor diet, late nights, or too many hours spent at a computer. They can also signify more serious health issues, which should receive medical attention. Try these massage techniques to rest the eyes and improve circulation.

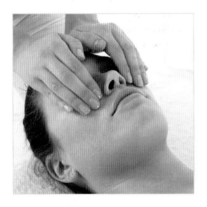

resting over the eyes This is great for relaxing the eyes. Rub your hands together vigorously until they feel warm. Cup your hands over your partner's eyes so that your heels rest on the forehead and your fingers over the cheeks. Bend your wrists to lift your palms away from the eyes. Simply rest. The warmth from your hands will help rejuvenate the eyes.

circling the temples Place your fingertips over the temples. Make a fairly large half-circle back toward the hairline so that you lift the skin. This stimulates the circulation round the eye area and is psychologically uplifting too. Repeat in several places over the temples, lifting your fingers at the end of each movement so as not to drag the skin.

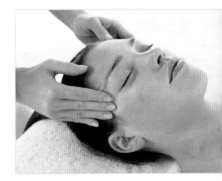

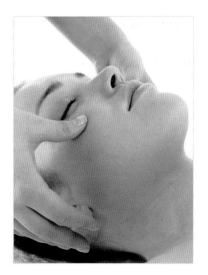

### thumb circling under the eyes

Lack of circulation is one cause of dark circles. Place your thumbs over the lower eye-socket ridge, just by the bridge of your partner's nose. Circle outward in small spirals toward the temples, taking care not to drag delicate skin. Repeat in several lines outward under the eyes to stimulate circulation to the muscles.

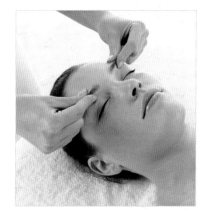

### squeezing the browline

Squeeze along the browline, tracing the arc of the eyebrows around to the temples. Begin by the nose and pinch firmly between your index fingers and thumbs. Repeat several times for tired eyes. This is great for relieving tension and brightening the eyes.

# Lower backache

Aches in the lower back can be due to poor posture and a sedentary lifestyle and contribute to shoulder and neck tension. Try these techniques to relax the muscles and improve overall posture. Always apply some general relaxing massage strokes first.

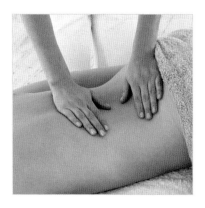

**palm pressure on the lower back** Place one hand, palm flat, over your partner's sacrum, the bony triangle at the base of the spine. Place the other hand over the muscles at the lower back, cupping your hand to avoid pressure on the spine. Stretch your palms away from each other without sliding over the skin. This gives the lower back muscles a good stretch. Repeat several times.

**forearm pressure on the lower back** Place your forearms facing each other diagonally over the lower back. Gradually slide over the muscles while applying pressure, so that one arm ends by the ribcage, and the other over the hip. This provides another good muscle stretch. Repeat the stroke by swapping the direction of your arms.

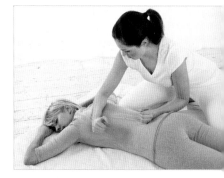

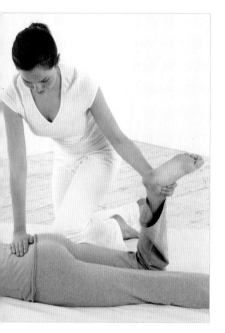

bending the legs With one hand on the body for support, slide your other hand under the ankle. Lift the lower leg and rotate, then slowly bend back and away from you toward the opposite hip. This strengthens the kidney meridian and is good for sciatica.

elbow pressure on the buttocks Locate GB 30, which is the point two-thirds of the way across the buttocks and one-third down. Press into the point with a rounded elbow, circling and kneading the muscles. If this is painful, circle around rather than over the point itself. Repeat on the other hip to stimulate energy circulation and for sciatica relief.

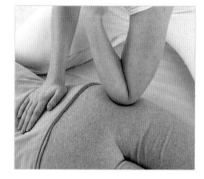

# Premenstrual syndrome (PMS)

Premenstrual syndrome can make you feel awful, ranging from emotionally irritable to having severe pain over the lower back and abdomen. Diet can help, but try these massage techniques too. Work gently, over a few days, to relieve pain and tension and promote blood flow.

circling the lower back Spread some warmed oil over your hands and effleurage your partner's lower back with long, slow, comforting strokes. Then circle over the lower back in a counterclockwise direction with one hand on top of the other. Use the pressure that feels best for your partner. The strokes will warm and relax the lower back muscles.

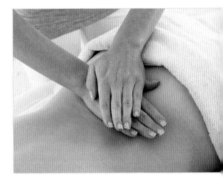

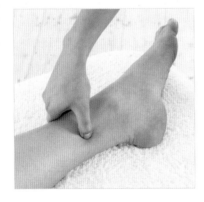

thumb pressure on the ankles Slide your thumb up the inner leg, about three finger-widths up from the ankle joint. Press behind the bone to find Sp 6, which may be very tender. If so, circle around the spot to ease the blood flow. Hold for a few moments, then release and circle again to relieve any tenderness.

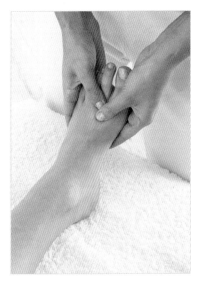

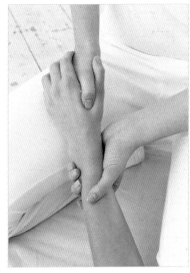

thumb pressure on the feet Find Li 3, which lies between the base of the big and first toes. Rub and circle over the point first if it feels tender, and then press in more deeply with your thumb. Begin slowly and increase your pressure, then hold for a few moments. This is a good point to stimulate the week before PMS may occur.

thumb pressure on the hands Place your thumb over LI 4, which lies in the web between the index finger and thumb. Reach up until you locate the point, pressing gently at first, and rub on the spot until it feels less tender. Then press in with your thumb, with your middle finger providing support from underneath. Hold for a few moments and then release. Repeat all the movements on the other side.

# Aching feet

Feet have to work hard bearing our weight. If you are standing up all day or wear high heels, your feet may really ache. A good massage at the end of the day with some peppermint foot cream should help, and is a lovely treat to give your partner. Firm pressure avoids any tickling.

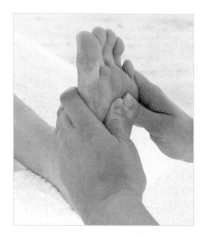

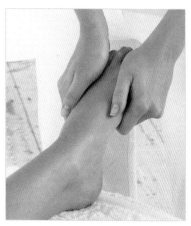

circling the soles of the feet
With your partner's legs raised, use your thumbs to circle over the soles of their feet. Circle, knead and press over the foot with the balls of your thumbs. Avoid pressure over the instep as this can be uncomfortable, but otherwise massage thoroughly until the feet feel softer.

squeezing the feet Place your hands on either side of the foot and squeeze. Then push one side of the foot upward while pulling down on the other side. Change direction several times to stimulate the circulation and get movement into the foot. This reduces stiffness and counteracts the effects of being on your feet for hours.

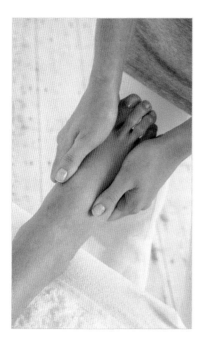

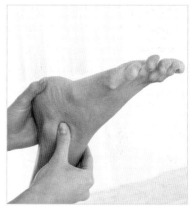

circling the ankles Circle the ankle joint with your thumb to stimulate the circulation and restore movement. Big, broad circles feel best; you can press and circle close in to the joint afterward. Encourage passive ankle movement while you are massaging, to help release any stiffness. Repeat all the movements on the other side.

thumb pressure on the feet Cup your hands around the foot so that your thumbs are over the top. Place them lengthways side by side and then slide them outward. Apply resistance with your fingers underneath. Repeat the movement in several lines, squeezing your partner's feet to relax the muscles.

# Stiff neck

For most people the area where they usually feel tension is in the neck and shoulders. A stiff neck can be the result of poor posture and a sedentary lifestyle and can lead to headaches, so try these massage techniques to relieve tension and relax the muscles.

kneading the shoulders Knead along the top of your partner's shoulders, beginning at the neck and working outward. Your fingers should rest over the shoulders while your thumbs knead the muscles. Press and circle over the muscles, paying attention to any tense spots. Where the muscles feel tender, reduce the amount of pressure and increase the breadth of your strokes.

circling the neck Place your thumbs on the muscles to the side of the spine, beside the prominent vertebra (C7) at the base of the neck. With your fingers resting over the shoulders, circle and press to relax the muscles, which in turn will relax the neck. This particular point is known as GV 14.

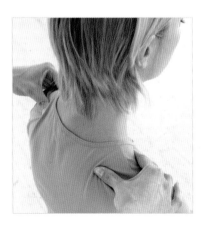

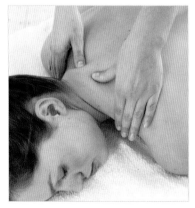

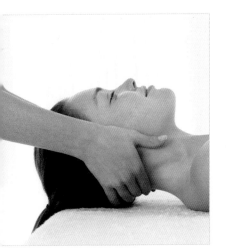

pulling the neck With your partner lying face upward, slide both hands under the neck and then cradle the base of the skull. Lift the head slightly and gently pull it back toward you so that you give the neck a stretch. This helps to ease neck tension and gives the feeling of lengthening the spine. Lower the head again very gently.

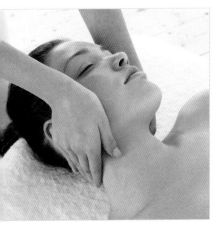

rocking the head Slide your hands under the neck and cradle the base of the skull. Turn the head to one side by pressing your hand flat against the neck, then turn it the other way with your other hand. Gently rock the head from side to side to encourage the neck and shoulder muscles to relax.

# Thinning hair

These massage techniques may help where hair growth is diminishing due to lack of circulation or stress. Massage increases the blood flow over the scalp and stimulates the hair follicles. In a healthy person, massage should stimulate hair growth over a period of weeks.

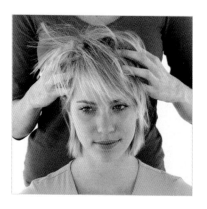
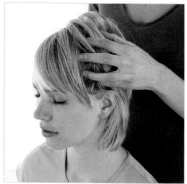

finger pressure on the scalp
Place the balls of your fingers and thumbs on your partner's scalp and make shampooing movements over the entire head. Work right through to the ends of the hair. Gentle tugging at the roots is helpful, too. Your fingers should slide over the scalp, applying firm pressure and encouraging movement of the hair. Be careful not to actually pull out any hair over thinning areas.

rotating over the scalp Place the fingers of one hand on the scalp, and the other hand on the head to provide support. Rotate over the scalp with the balls of your fingers and thumb. Spread your fingers so that your hand maintains the same shape throughout. Rotate and circle on the spot without sliding over the skin, to stimulate circulation.

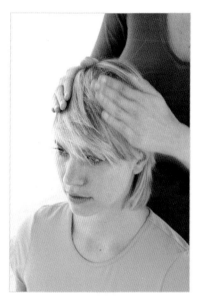 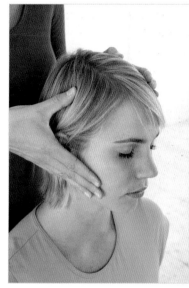

rubbing the scalp Rub vigorously
over the head with the flat of your hand,
placing your other hand on the head for
support. Your movements should provide
friction over the scalp as you rub back
and forth. Work small areas at a time very
thoroughly and you should feel some
warmth beneath your hand. Work
sensitively where the hair is thinning.

thumb circling the scalp
Supporting the head with one hand, circle
over the scalp with your other hand. Use
small spiralling movements with the tip of
your thumb to stimulate the scalp. Work
gently but thoroughly over thinning
areas, and especially where the hairline is
receding. Applying some nourishing hair
oil may also help.

# Cellulite

What is commonly known as cellulite, or orange-peel skin, usually involves fluid retention and congestion of the tissues. Along with massage, diet and exercise play important roles. Massage sensitively as these areas are often tender. Repeat on a daily basis.

### kneading the thighs and buttocks
Kneading is good for clearing congestion, but be careful because the pressure can be painful. Work over your partner's thigh and buttock area, pressing into the muscles with your thumbs and rolling back with your fingers. The hands should work alternately and establish rhythmic movements. The addition of cleansing essential oils may help.

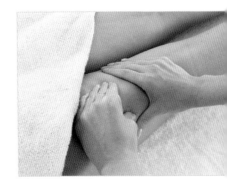

### heel pressure on the thighs
Massage along the thigh muscles with the heels of your hands, working up to the hip. Apply enough pressure to be effective, but not painful. Work up over the thigh with both hands using long, alternate strokes, or use both hands together for greater pressure. Avoid any massage over the inner thigh.

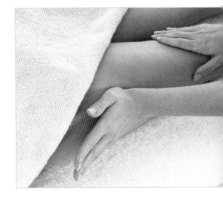

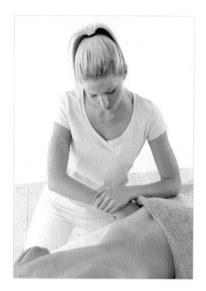

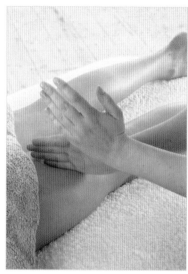

knuckle pressure on the
buttocks and legs Form your hand
into a loose fist and massage congested
areas with your knuckles. This can be
quite effective, but be careful where there
is a lack of muscle tone. Circle and knead
on the spot to increase the circulation,
but keep to fleshy areas. Avoid massage
directly over the bones or inner thigh.

percussion on the thighs Use
your hands to hack up and down the
thigh to increase circulation. Your wrists
should be kept loose and body contact
made with your little fingers. Your
movements need to be sharp and light to
achieve the traditional hacking sound. You
can also use other percussion movements,
such as pummelling and cupping, to
stimulate the local circulation. Repeat all
the movements on the other leg.

# Colds and flu

Colds can be a sign that your immunity is low, and flu definitely requires bed rest and medical advice. To ease the symptoms of an ordinary cold, try these massage techniques. At the same time reduce your stress levels and follow a healthy diet.

### thumb pressure on the hands

Place your thumb over the web between your partner's index finger and thumb. Locate LI 4, which lies just between the bones, and press with the tip of your thumb. At the same time squeeze underneath with your middle finger to provide some resistance. The spot may be painful, so approach it gently. Hold for a few moments, and repeat over several days to help reduce excess heat.

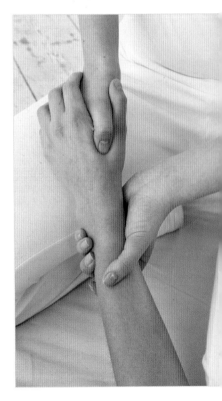

### CAUTION

Do not use point LI 4 during pregnancy.

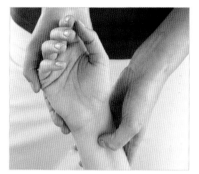

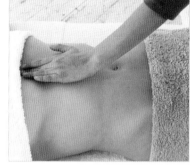

**thumb pressure on the wrists**
Locate P6, which lies centrally between the tendons, two and a half finger-widths above the wrist. Press with the tip of your thumb, holding the forearm underneath for resistance, for a general tonic or to reduce heat. Press and hold the point for a few moments, then release and repeat the actions on the other wrist.

**finger pressure on the chest**
Locate CV 17, which is on the breastbone, midpoint between the nipples. Press the point with the ball of your finger, hold for a few moments, then circle on the spot. This is very good to help ease breathing and relax emotional tension in the chest. Repeat over several days to improve the symptoms.

**circling the head** The symptoms of stressed muscles and those of flu can sometimes become confused. Instead of curling up (a natural instinct when you feel ill), try massaging around the forehead, scalp, and neck with small fingertip circles. This can often help the body to return to normal and give you the opportunity for recovery before illness strikes.

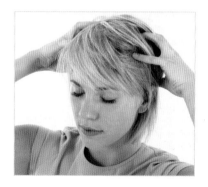

# Digestive problems

Problems with digestion can be caused by poor diet and lifestyle, lack of exercise, and stress. Chronic problems need qualified attention, but try these massage techniques to relieve general discomfort. Also, review your eating habits and set aside time for proper meals.

palm pressure on the legs Your partner should lie on the floor, legs turned slightly inward. With one hand on their body for support, "walk" down the side of the crest of the muscles, following the stomach meridian. Press with your palm, release and continue pressing steadily and evenly the length of the leg. Avoid any pressure over the knee.

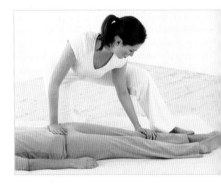

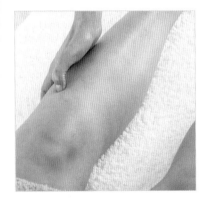

thumb pressure on the legs
Locate St 36, which lies in the depression by the shinbone, three finger-widths below the knee. Massage and circle over the point with the ball of your thumb to improve digestion. Then press the point directly, hold for a few moments and release. This is a good constitutional point to massage from time to time. Repeat the movements on the other leg.

## effleurage on the abdomen

A relaxed abdomen can aid digestion. Rub a little oil between your hands and circle in a clockwise direction over your partner's abdomen. The strokes should be made with the flats of your hands, avoiding too much pressure. The aim is to relax and soothe so that the natural digestive processes can take place.

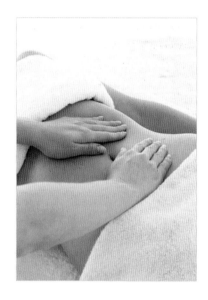

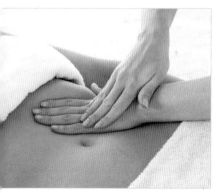

## palm pressure on the abdomen

Place the flat of your hand just beneath the ribcage and the other hand on top for support. Press very gently as your partner breathes out. Relax your pressure and try again, each time coordinating as your partner exhales. Repeat on the other side to encourage relaxation, but make sure the pressure causes no discomfort.

# Anxiety

Anxiety can prevent people from functioning properly. Chronic cases need specialized support, but for temporary situations, try some relaxing techniques to reduce mental agitation. Fears are usually about what might happen, so use massage to stay in the present moment.

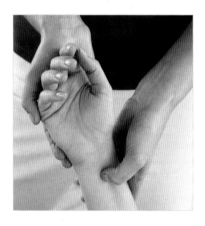

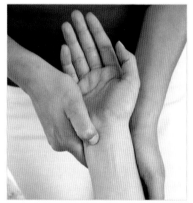

thumb pressure on the wrist

Support your partner's arm with one hand, and locate P6 between the tendons, two and a half finger-widths above the wrist. Place your thumb over the point and press gently with the ball, hold for a few moments and then release. Used together with the following point, this is very useful whenever your partner feels anxious or stressed.

thumb pressure on the wrist

Find the depression in a line down from the inside of the little finger, just below the wrist. This point is H7. Place your thumb close in to the bone and press it with the tip. Hold for a few moments, then release to provide support and reduce anxiety. Use this in conjunction with the point described above. Repeat the actions on the other wrist.

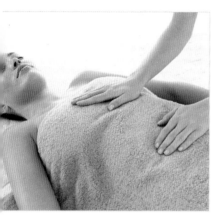

resting With your partner lying face up and covered for comfort, breathe calmly, empty your mind and place one hand on the lower abdomen and the other over the chest. Let your hands rise and fall with your partner's breath. This calms the emotions and encourages relaxed breathing, which becomes shallow when we are stressed.

effleurage on the back Rub some warmed oil over your hands and effleurage over the back with broad, sweeping strokes. Work from the lower back up to the shoulders, where your hands should separate and return down the sides of the ribs. Repeat slowly to reassure your partner, then end by effleuraging over the lower back and legs, finishing at the feet.

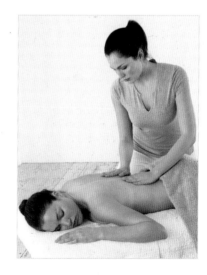

# Colic

This can be a distressing condition in the first few months of a baby's life, which can leave you feeling helpless. Try the following movements between episodes to help calm your baby. Staying calm yourself stops your baby from picking up on your anxiety.

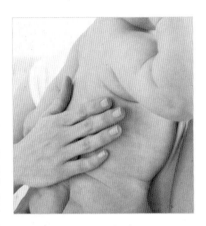

circling the back Just the gentle reassurance of your touch can help. With your baby in an upright position to help ease any gas, make broad, comforting circles over the back. Massage especially to help ease the abdomen. The circles should be counterclockwise with whole-hand contact. Simply the warmth of your hand will help.

bending the legs Gently bend the leg at the knee and bring the thigh slowly toward the chest. Do not overstretch or exert any pressure. This helps to ease pressure on the abdomen. Repeat the movement several times with each leg, and stop as soon as you feel any resistance. This is best done when your baby is feeling comfortable.

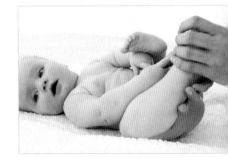

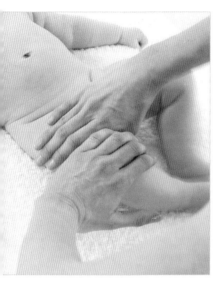

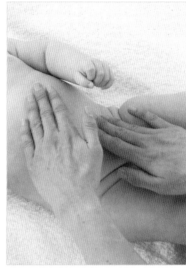

**effleurage on the legs** Rub a little oil over your fingers and gently stroke up the legs from ankles to thighs, avoiding any pressure over the knees. Massage on the thighs is good for the circulation and may help to ease the discomfort of colic. Stroke toward the abdomen, then brush lightly down the legs, keeping to a soothing rhythm.

**effleurage on the abdomen** Rub a little oil over your fingers and effleurage gently over the abdomen. Follow the direction of the large intestine, and circle clockwise in soothing strokes. This is best done on a regular basis to help keep the abdomen relaxed. Use light strokes with the flats of your fingers.

# Teething

Teething is a painful time and is hard to watch when your baby is in distress. Some gentle massage over the gums can help improve the local circulation. Massage is not only soothing in itself, but can provide a welcome distraction. Massage on a regular basis.

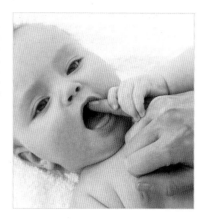

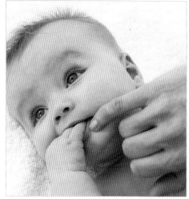

circling the gums Massage very gently and with care over your baby's gums. Using the tip of your little finger, make very small circles and massage as high up the gums as you can. Each movement over the upper gums should end in an upward direction; downward for the lower gums. Do not massage where there is inflammation.

circling the mouth Try circling movements over the gums, this time working gently on the face. Press and circle gently with the tip of your little finger to stimulate the circulation and drainage. Work around the mouth, pressing gently against the gums. The strokes should end in an upward direction over the upper gums, and downward over the lower gums.

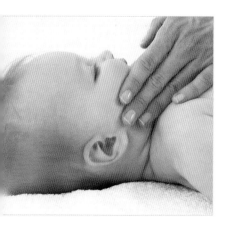

circling the jaw Circle very gently around the angle of the jaw, to increase the circulation. Use your fingertips in soothing movements, using slightly more pressure as you circle back toward the ears. Keep your fingertips flat so that they do not dig in, and lift the skin slightly as you stroke.

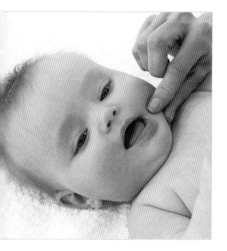

squeezing the jaw Use the tips of your fingers and thumbs to lightly squeeze around the angle of the jaw. As you squeeze, lift the muscles slightly so that it becomes almost a soft, pinching movement. Lifting rather than pressing helps to ease the pressure and stimulates the local circulation. It can also be made into a little game.

# Repetitive strain injury (RSI)

Working on computer keyboards, or at any activity where you constantly repeat small movements, can result in severe symptoms over time. Keep your fingers and hands supple through daily massage and exercise to provide a variety of movement for your muscles.

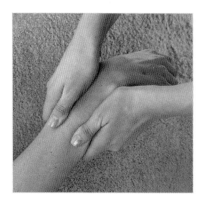

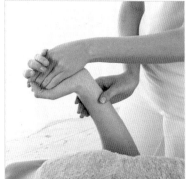

squeezing the wrists Place your thumbs together in the center of your partner's forearm, with your fingers cupped around the wrist. Apply pressure with the length of your thumbs and slowly draw them out to your fingers. This works best without oil so that you can squeeze the muscles more tightly. Increasing the circulation and improving drainage are vital to minimizing strain.

rotating the wrists Grasp the hand and rotate at the wrist to maintain joint mobility. As long as there is no discomfort, try to achieve as great a range of movement as possible. Strain arises from repeating the same movements over and over again, so maintaining flexibility is very important.

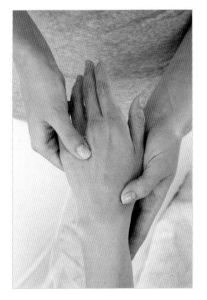

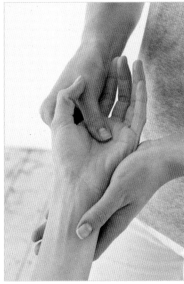

squeezing the hands Spread a little oil over your hands and reach up between your partner's fingers, with your thumb on top and middle finger underneath. Squeeze firmly between finger and thumb as you draw down between the tendons. Repeat this over both hands, pressing and circling to release any tension.

circling the palms Supporting the hand from underneath for resistance, circle and press over the palm with your thumb. Use firm pressure as you circle and squeeze over the muscles and joints. Remember to massage the fleshy pads at the thumb and side of the hand. Circle carefully around the base of the finger joints until the muscles start to relax.

# Painful joints

It is very important to maintain mobility by stimulating the circulation. Massage should not be done when the joints are inflamed, and great care should be taken not to cause pain. Diet is an important factor in preventing the build up of waste products which may irritate the body.

squeezing the thighs To improve the circulation and drainage, work above but not over your partner's joints. Apply a little oil to your hands, then squeeze over the thigh muscles, draining toward the hips. Make sure there is no pressure on the knee joint, and use a support if necessary. Squeeze using whole-hand contact to cover the length of the thigh.

circling the shoulders As long as the joint is not currently inflamed, cup your fingers around the ball of your partner's shoulder and circle around (but not over) the joint with your thumbs. Use broad circles, sweeping away from the joint. Some warming oil may also be helpful to soothe and stimulate the circulation.

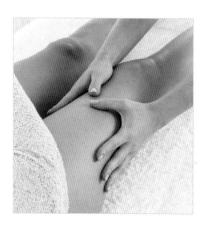

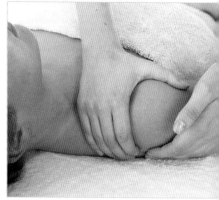

## thumb pressure on the fingers
Use your thumbs to press around (but not directly over or under) the finger joint. Stop if there is any pain. Press and circle gently, working close in to the bones. Bend the finger as you massage, if this is comfortable, to increase the circulation and encourage mobility. Gentle passive exercise is always helpful.

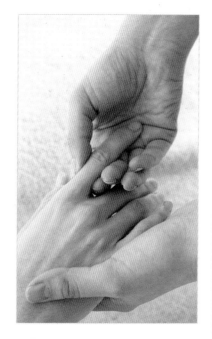

## rotating the fingers
Do this only if the joints are not inflamed. Grasp a finger, pull gently, and rotate. Try to get as much movement as possible. Rotate the finger in wide circles and then try a bicycling motion. A few minutes' daily passive exercise of the joints helps to reduce stiffness over time. Repeat all the movements on both hands.

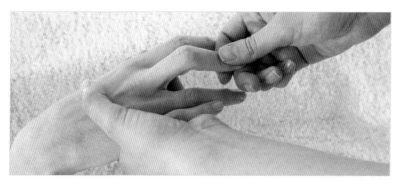

# Earache

Earache can have a variety of causes. It can be very painful and in acute or prolonged episodes may require medical attention. However, for mild complaints these decongestive massage techniques may help. Repeat the strokes as often as necessary.

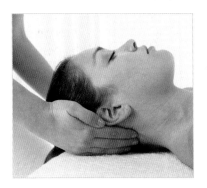

circling the ears Use the tips of your fingers to gently massage the area behind your partner's ears. Start your circles at the hairline and gradually move toward the ears. Of particular benefit is the area closest in. The direction of the circles, however, is away from the ear itself. Check that the pressure is not causing discomfort and continue gently for several minutes.

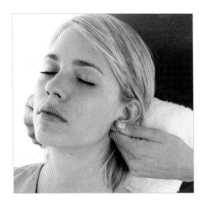

squeezing the ears Lightly pinch along the inside of the ears with your thumbs and index fingers, squeezing in several lines as the movements follow the shape of the ears. As you reach the entrance to the ear canal, lift the earlobes and gently tug them. Gradually work in closer to the ear canal, squeezing and kneading all the time.

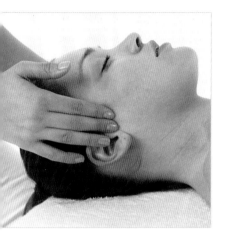

finger pressure on the jaw Ask your partner to relax or drop their jaw. Press your fingertips close in to the angle of the jaw, then continue massaging around the area, working toward the thickening of the entrance to the ear canal. Knead and press gently around the area until your partner feels some relief. Keep checking the jaw is released.

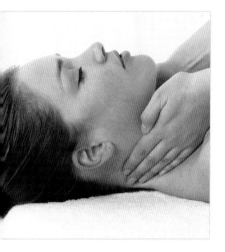

circling over the neck Place the fingertips of both hands flat over the neck muscles, just below the earlobes. Make slow half-circles back toward the spine, moving the skin as you do so. The area may feel a little puffy or tender. Work slowly and repetitively for several minutes to increase drainage. This should help the feeling of being "blocked."

# Poor circulation

This may result in cold hands and feet and can generally be helped by a little exercise and some massage techniques to promote circulation and increase energy flow throughout the body. Poor circulation has different causes and more serious conditions require medical advice.

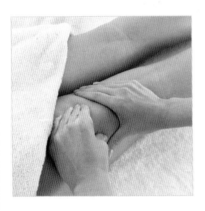

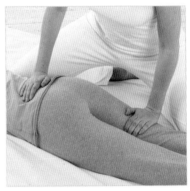

kneading the legs Where the circulation is poor, the skin may be cooler to the touch or a different color from the surrounding body area. Knead firmly to increase the circulation over muscular areas, particularly the thighs and buttocks. Press in with your thumbs and roll with your fingers until you notice a visible difference.

palm pressure on the arms or legs Position yourself at your partner's side, hold one hand on the body for support and use the other palm to "walk" over the arms or legs, depending on where the problem lies. Position your hand, press, hold, and release, working in lines along the meridians. Work more gently over any joints and repeat several times. Stretching and pulling will also help to improve energy flow.

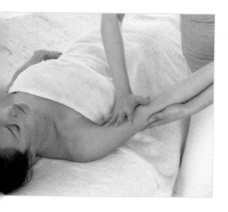

rubbing the arms Use the flat of your hand to rub down the heart meridian on the little-finger side of the inner arm. Work from the armpit down to the little finger. Then firmly pinch and squeeze the length of the arm and squeeze the finger. End by pulling over the fingertip quickly with a little snap. This helps to promote the circulation.

thumb pressure on the legs
Locate Sp 6, which is the point three finger-widths above the ankle joint, just behind the bone. This is good for the circulation and for providing a general tonic. Begin gently since this point can be quite tender. Press with the ball of your thumb, hold, and then release. Circle around the point as a softer alternative. Repeat all movements on the other side.

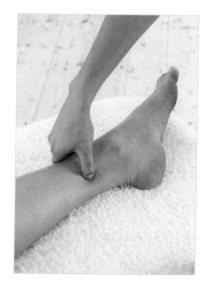

CAUTION

Do not use point Sp 6 during pregnancy.

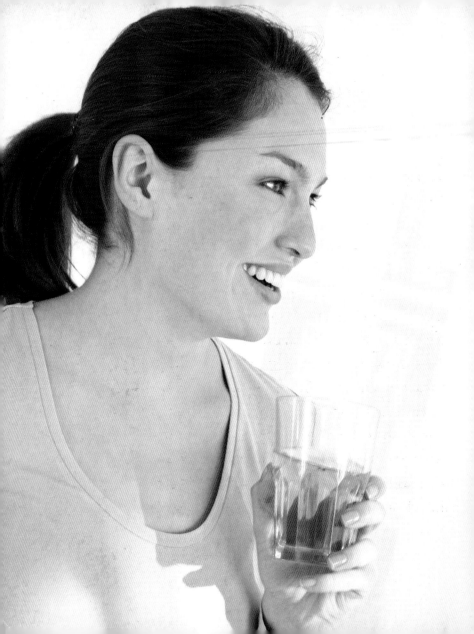

# Lifestyle tips

Massage forms just part of the framework of keeping body and mind healthy. The tips that follow are tasters of some of the other ways in which you can take responsibility for your own well-being. As you try them out, you may feel drawn to exploring some of the approaches in greater depth. Some work well in certain situations or for certain personalities, while at other times or for other people another method may appeal. Any or all of these approaches complement massage. Feeling helpless makes any problem worse, whereas making a choice for a positive lifestyle is actually more interesting and a lot more fun!

# Stress

The most common reaction to massage is a feeling of intense relaxation, and this simple word covers a multitude of benefits. However, an absence of relaxation, or the presence of prolonged stress, can have a negative impact on our health, self-esteem, and quality of life.

## The "fight or flight" response

A certain amount of stress is good. It challenges and motivates us to be creative. Acute stress stimulates the sympathetic nervous system, and the adrenal glands secrete chemicals that speed up the metabolic processes, providing the energy to respond to danger; this is popularly known as the "fight or flight" response. Short-term responses are an increase in heart rate and respiration, dilated pupils, and sweating. The increase in energy promotes muscular activity and enables us to take appropriate physical action. Resources are temporarily diverted from functions less useful for crisis situations, such as reproduction, digestion, and sleep. These reactions to stimuli are natural responses, which our bodies are well able to deal with.

It is the effects of prolonged, chronic stress that can be debilitating and have serious consequences for our health. When we are constantly stimulated and on the alert, our resources become depleted. More hormones are released than the body can deal with, resulting in both physical and mental exhaustion. Switching off becomes difficult, and it is this constant low-level stress that is dangerous and needs to be addressed.

## Reversing stress through massage

Responses to stress are individual, and so is tolerance. What may be exciting for one person is stressful for another. Sensitive individuals may be much more susceptible. However, our modern lifestyles with their accent on achievement and material values, overstimulation, poor diet, lack of exercise, and poor sleep quality play a large part in our ability to cope. It is all too easy to lose that natural healthy balance.

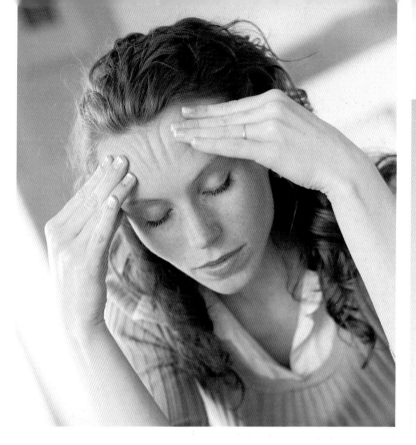

Fortunately, once you actually start to deal with stress, the damage can be reversed. Massage is a fantastic tool, with its physical benefits of speeding up the elimination of metabolic wastes, such as the hormones produced by stress. Of equal benefit is its ability to relax the mind, inducing a sense of

*Stress can have a debilitating impact on our quality of life. Massage provides a great tool for reducing its effects.*

confidence and well-being. And once you have experienced true, deep relaxation, the pursuit of a positive, balanced lifestyle becomes a way of life.

## STRESS-BUSTING TIPS

Here are some tips for dealing with stress in the short term. However, a long-term approach is going to require a little work to achieve permanent change.

▶ Change what you can. Do not let situations become chronic. There are external factors that you can alter and you should do this as soon as possible.

▶ For external factors that you cannot change you need to alter your reaction.

▶ Take a deep breath before reacting to a situation. You may find that you come out with a different more measured response.

▶ Do everything in moderation to reduce the rollercoaster extremes of highs and lows.

▶ Get plenty of exercise in the fresh air. A healthy body deals better with stress.

▶ Cut down on salty and sugary snacks and food.

▶ Reduce the usual props, such as caffeine, alcohol, cigarettes, or drugs. They make you feel worse in the long term.

▶ Find new healthy props to give you energy, such as fresh foods, a makeover, good music, or a relaxing bath with essential oils.

▶ Prioritize. Deal with one stressful situation at a time.

▶ Surround yourself with positive, uplifting people.

▶ Learn from your mistakes.

▶ Take time out for your needs, without feeling guilty about it.

▶ Help someone else. It will put your own problems into perspective.

▶ Get help if you cannot cope. This is a positive thing to do.

▶ Make getting an early night a regular feature. You cannot solve problems when you are tired.

▶ Have more fun—laughter keeps us healthy and makes problems seem easier to overcome.

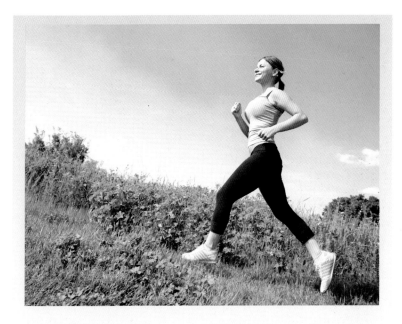

▶ Make your relationships more positive. See the best in people.

▶ If you cannot get regular massage, make up a daily self-massage routine and stick to it.

▶ Express your emotions in a positive way. Bottling them up inside can lead to disaster.

▶ Listen to your heart rather than your head.

*Regular exercise helps to keep mind and body healthy and to reduce the negative effects of stress.*

▶ Be your own best friend. Give yourself credit when you do well, or simply for trying, if things don't work out. A mental pat on the back works wonders.

# Relaxation

Relaxation is the way the body recovers from exertion, whether physical or mental. These processes are governed by the parasympathetic nervous system (see page 18) and help to maintain internal balance. Relaxation is an active rather than passive state.

It can include recreation, but often we relax our bodies while continuing to stimulate our minds. True relaxation refreshes the whole of us and gives us a new perspective on life. There are different techniques to suit different people, which may require some practice at first.

## How to do progressive relaxation

Lie or sit in a comfortable position. Take note of any areas of your body that feel tense or uncomfortable. Then physically tense and relax each part of you in turn, beginning at the feet and working up to the head. Relax for a few minutes and breathe calmly. Then work back down the body, moving each part in turn until you reach the feet.

*True relaxation requires practice and a little effort, but experiment with different techniques to find a method to suit you.*

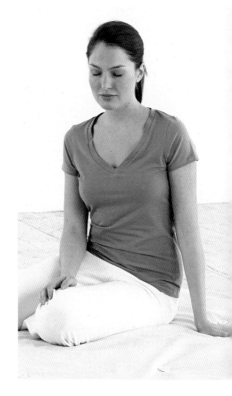

# Visualization

Some people can visualize easily, although it is not for everyone. Visualization is a way of channeling mental energy into something positive: you create an ideal situation in your mind. Include as much sensory information as possible so that it becomes a real experience, and recall the image or feelings that you experienced whenever you need to. Visualizations may be guided by someone else, so that you can let go and put everything into the experience.

## How to do a visualization

Find a quiet place where you are comfortable. Some music may help you relax. Let go of everyday problems and breathe calmly. Imagine yourself somewhere pleasant, such as a country field. Experience all the sights, sounds, smells, and colors. Then start walking to the top of a nearby hill, sit down, look around, and remember that feeling.

# Sleep

Good-quality sleep is vital for the body to repair itself after the day's exertions. Too often we experience broken sleep, or have difficulty switching off mentally. People vary in the amount of sleep they need, and worrying about lack of sleep only increases anxiety. Establishing a wind-down routine can help, or try the occasional catnap to catch up.

## SLEEPING TIPS

► Avoid caffeine or a heavy meal just before going to bed.

► Have a warm bath or shower a few hours before bed and apply some relaxing oils.

► Let go of the day's problems, which you can do nothing about now and will deal with tomorrow.

► Make your bedroom a relaxation zone with soft lighting and soothing music.

► Put a drop of essential oil under your pillow.

► Think of someone or something nice. Relax.

# Meditation, oils, and herbs

Meditation calms the mind and emotions. Techniques are often linked to a spiritual tradition, but can be practiced on their own. It is a good idea to get some guidance from an experienced teacher. Techniques vary from emptying the mind to focusing on the breath or an object or sound.

## How to meditate

Find a comfortable position where you can be quiet. Breathe calmly and relax your body. Focus your attention on your breath as you breathe in and out, but do not try and breathe in any special way. Let go of any thoughts that come into your mind and do not get emotionally involved. Try this for ten minutes every day. Eventually you will find that you are calmer.

## Oils

Essential oils can be used to help relaxation. They can be applied in a body lotion, a bath oil, or used to fragrance a room. Use only natural oils and avoid synthetic preparations. Essential-oil molecules can trigger a process whereby electrical impulses are relayed to the brain, having a positive effect on mood. Choose therapeutic oils that you like (see pages 388–389). Put a drop or two on a tissue for emergencies, but *never* use them directly on the skin. Try bergamot, lavender, or geranium to lift your mood.

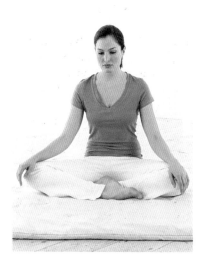

*Most meditation techniques involve sitting in a meditative posture. With practice you can achieve peace of mind.*

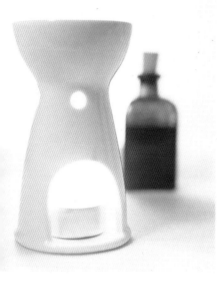

*Essential oils and herbs can aid relaxation. Make choosing them and their preparation part of the therapeutic process.*

# Herbs

The use of herbs goes back to early civilizations and in many traditions formed part of the system of medical treatment. For therapeutic use you must find a qualified herbalist, but some herbs are safe to use on their own. Teas can be made from fresh or dried herbs and used to help relaxation. Containing no caffeine, herbal teas are excellent to take during the day, after a meal or to help you wind down in the evening before sleep.

### How to make a herbal infusion

Prepare a warmed pot. To make an infusion to aid relaxation, add one heaped teaspoonful of dried herbs such as chamomile, lemon balm, or lime flowers (if using fresh herbs, double the amount). Add boiling water and allow to steep for about ten minutes. You can add a spoonful of honey according to taste, if you wish. To aid digestion, prepare a pot of peppermint tea and drink after your meal; for improved concentration and mental focus, try a pot of rosemary tea.

### How to fragrance a room

Place some oils in a diffuser. Use a few drops of your favorite essential oil or try equal numbers of drops of up to three oils. The scent should fragrance the room. Do not leave the diffuser unattended. Oils can also be added to a base of water in a candle burner, which should be placed on an even surface and not left unattended. Air the room afterward to avoid saturation, and do not use around children or pets.

# Positive attitude

Stress is an individual response to a situation that you may or may not be able to do anything about. If you can, do something to resolve the problem, which will instantly make you feel better. If you can't, try to change something about your response, which will alleviate the pressure.

For example, if you normally get very emotional or flustered, take a deep breath and count to ten before responding; you may come out with something different. Rather than getting into a confrontation, remove yourself physically from the situation until things are calmer, and do something else. Don't be a doormat. If you normally bottle up your emotions, let them out in a positive way and do something constructive. If you like to be in control, ease off a little. If you prefer to go with the flow, take charge for a change.

Once you become stressed, it is easy to become anxious about the next trigger, so try to stay positive and simply enjoy the present moment. Look at problems as opportunities to use your ingenuity, or to develop hidden qualities within yourself. Focusing on the here and now is a great way of changing your usual response.

## Learning opportunity

When you encounter a problem or difficulty in a relationship, take a step back and ask yourself what you need to learn from the situation. Try to be as objective as possible. Then try finding an alternative solution based on what you observe. It only needs one person to change their response to turn a situation around.

## Seeing the best

If you find something or someone difficult to deal with, try listing their good qualities for a change. Look through rose-tinted glasses and you may be surprised by what you find. Try and connect with the positive points. Then try the same exercise on yourself. We are often hardest of all on ourselves.

## Positive language

Practice being positive by only using positive language for a day. You may be

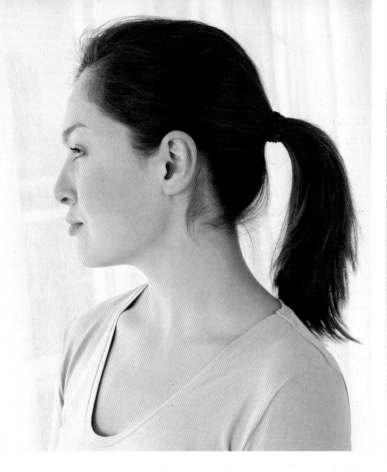

surprised at how negative language can affect your thoughts and reactions and stop you from trying something new. Negative connotations stick. Try and approach everything and everyone afresh, with an open mind.

*Stress can be eased by how we respond to situations. Forget familiar patterns and you may be surprised by the results.*

# Diet

The body is truly amazing and carries out tissue and cell repair on a daily basis. Every cell needs proper nourishment and a healthy environment to thrive—and that part is up to us. When we are busy, a balanced diet is often compromised and we end up running on empty.

Lack of decent nutrition adds to our stress levels and affects our ability to cope and think clearly. It also shows up in skin problems, lacklustre hair and nails, chronic low-level aches and pains, or a susceptibility to infection.

To keep healthy, do a little research to find out what good nutrition really involves, and keep a close eye on the ingredients in the food you eat. Try cutting down on stimulants such as caffeine and alcohol, which ultimately deplete your energy. Reduce your intake of salty foods, because salt promotes water retention in the tissues. And try cutting down on sugar, which provides a breeding ground for viruses and unhealthy cells. Processed foods lack nutritional value, so spend a little time creating healthy snacks of your own.

*Small changes can yield big results. Try increasing the amount of water you drink and see how much better you feel.*

And make time not only to enjoy your food, but for proper digestion too. Eating late at night can cause sleeplessness, so eat earlier or have lighter meals.

We generally know what we *should* be eating, so what does it take to change? Try the following suggestions.

## Cleansing

A good inner cleanser for the day is a cup of plain boiled water with a fresh slice of lemon. Add a little honey if you need to.

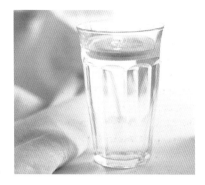

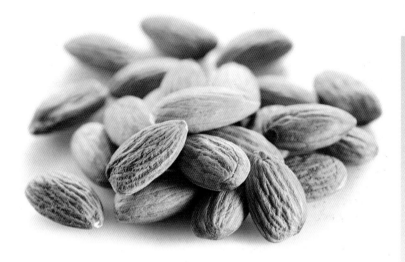

Drink this first thing and see how much fresher you feel. Then try substituting at least one regular tea or coffee every day for a cup of herbal or green tea.

## Natural foods

Too much salty food is unhealthy, so try eating foods that have a good natural sodium and potassium balance. One of the best is celery, so chop up some organic celery as a snack. Almonds are also great, and an excellent food for the brain (but they can be toxic if eaten in excess); eat just a few on a regular basis.

*Good nutrition helps our bodies to function properly. Eat healthy snacks through the day to maintain high energy levels.*

## Acidity

Too much acidity can cause problems for the body, and in particular may contribute to joint pain. Try and balance your diet with alkaline foods, which means plenty of fresh vegetables. Growing your own on a small scale is fun. Try bean sprouts in glass jars, or salad herbs in a windowbox. That way your food is vibrant and fresh.

# Exercise

Exercise is good for the body. It improves the circulation, which means that the cells are well supplied with nutrients and the muscles with oxygen. It keeps the heart healthy and lowers blood pressure. It also improves drainage of the tissues through the removal of metabolic waste.

The lymph system, which helps to transport waste products, is stimulated by muscular activity. Through movement the joints are kept flexible, injuries heal faster, and a combination of fresh air and exercise produces clearer thinking and glowing skin. Moderate exposure to sunlight stimulates the production of vitamin D, which is important for maintaining good eyesight.

Finding time to exercise is vital, especially with increasing hours spent in sedentary pursuits. Exercise can be creative or formal, social, or solitary, or simply part of another activity. As with all things, moderation is the key, and exercise should be enjoyable rather than a chore. Beneficial exercise uses as many muscle groups as possible, without putting undue stress on the joints. Swimming is a great example. Regular daily exercise that you enjoy is something you will stick to, and

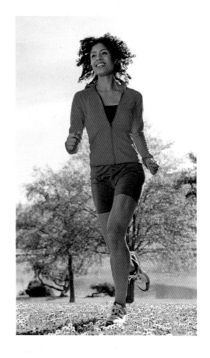

*Fresh air and exercise are a great combination. The more effort you put into it the greater the benefits you will feel.*

becomes even better once you see the results. If you are out of shape, get a health check first and always get first-class instruction. Try the following exercise suggestions.

## Mind and body exercise

Use exercise to promote the mind–body balance by taking up a discipline that addresses all aspects. Yoga or martial arts are ideal, not only for promoting physical health, but for calming the mind and emotions. With continued study, they will increase your self-knowledge and independence.

## Informal exercise

Exercise can be anything that gets you moving. Try walking briskly home from work for a change, with your arms swinging to help your lungs. Be more active when you exercise your pet. Do some bold planting in the garden. Take up dancing. Exercise can be something that you do as part of another activity, and then it feels more like fun.

## Stationary exercise

If you are not mobile for some reason, exercise is still important. Move as much as you can either sitting or lying down. Rotate your joints or pump your limbs

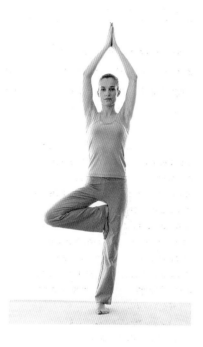

*Yoga is perfect for building strength and flexibility and improving posture. It can also help you develop a more positive outlook.*

up and down. The more you do, the easier it gets. Stretches are good. Yawning gets oxygen to the lungs. This is equally important if you are recovering from injury. The more you do to help your body, the more benefits you will feel.

# The after-effects of massage

So what can you expect from massage? What happens afterward? The physical effects of massage are improved circulation and drainage, increased flexibility of the joints, stimulation of the central nervous system and of the organs via the reflex points.

The skin generally improves as a result of the boost to peripheral circulation. And the immune system benefits due to increased drainage. The central nervous system is generally calmed, which produces a reduction in mental tension, soothes the emotions and generates positive well-being. Self-esteem is enhanced, together with an improved body image. Energy flow is stimulated, which results in better health. Thinking and perspective are enhanced and, through the focus on the senses, the mind and body feel better connected.

## Immediate and long-term effects

These processes can be quite pronounced the first time round. The muscles may ache a little afterward due to stimulation, or the recipient may feel a bit light-headed. This is usually due to changes in the blood pressure after lying down, so the best solution is to wait, roll over, and get up slowly. The recipient may feel really tired, again due to the body processes taking place, so the best option is to rest quietly for about an hour afterward and drink plenty of water.

Once massage becomes a regular feature, the cumulative benefits include better overall health, less stiffness, and greater flexibility, with an improved ability to deal with everyday situations. There also seems to be a more positive outlook on life.

## The benefits of giving and receiving

The benefits of any shared experience or activity bring two people closer. Massage is doubly rewarding because it concerns a special kind of emotional

*Massage on a regular basis provides real benefits, such as increased circulation, flexibility, self-esteem, and mental calm.*

communication that involves more than words. It is an unconditional form of giving and acceptance, offering the recipient a wonderful opportunity simply to rest and recharge.

Giving massage is calming, soothing, and improves relationships. As your techniques get better, so will your confidence, and it feels wonderful to develop such a therapeutic gift. Keep within your limits and do not overstretch your current reserves, allowing yourself some personal time to rebalance afterward.

Massage is positive, fascinating and an ideal way to spend quality time: an open-ended journey leading to unexpected destinations.

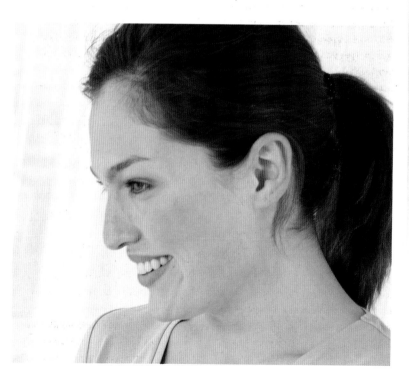

# Essential oil guide

Essential oils are aromatic volatile oils extracted from the roots, bark, stalks, leaves, fruit, and flowers of plants and trees. Their scents are therapeutic and have differing effects on the body, mind, and emotions. The oils are concentrated and should always be diluted and *never* applied directly to the skin.

Great care should be taken with them around children and animals. Essential oils are used in many bath and cosmetic preparations. For home use, they are great as room fragrancers (see pages 378–379) or can be added in mild dilutions to massage oil.

For massage, add up to four drops of essential oil to 2 teaspoons (10 ml) of vegetable oil (see pages 32–33). Choose natural essential oils of therapeutic grade from a reputable supplier. Due to environmental concerns, they should be ethically sourced.

## SUITABLE ESSENTIAL OILS

| NAME | QUALITIES | HOW TO USE |
| --- | --- | --- |
| Lemon (*Citrus limon*) | Uplifting | Good for oily skin, fatigue (Note: do not use on skin exposed to direct sunlight) |
| Grapefruit (*Citrus paradisi*) | Uplifting | Good for congested skin, nervous exhaustion |
| Bergamot (*Citrus bergamia*) | Uplifting | Good for spots, depression (Note: do not use on skin exposed to direct sunlight) |
| Neroli (*Citrus aurantium* var. *amara*) | A luxury oil; uplifting | Good for wrinkles, anxiety, shock (Note: do not use on skin exposed to direct sunlight; use sparingly) |

| | | |
|---|---|---|
| Eucalyptus (*Eucalyptus radiata*) | Stimulating | Use as a room fragrancer for respiratory problems |
| Tea tree (*Melaleuca alternifolia*) | Stimulating | Use as a room fragrancer for infections, colds and flu |
| Lavender (*Lavandula angustifolia*) | Calming | Good for allergies, nervous tension |
| Peppermint (*Mentha piperita*) | Stimulating | Good for foot massage, headaches (Note: too strong for a general body oil) |
| Chamomile (*Anthemis nobilis*) | Calming | Good for sensitive skin, insomnia |
| Rosemary (*Rosmarinus officinalis*) | Stimulating | Good for greasy skin, mental fatigue (Note: do not use in pregnancy, with epilepsy or high blood pressure) |
| Geranium (*Pelargonium graveolens*) | Balancing | Good for mature skin, stress (Note: use sparingly) |
| Ylang-ylang (*Cananga odorata* var. *genuina*) | Relaxing | Good for skin care, nervous tension, frustration (Note: use sparingly) |
| Jasmine (*Jasminum grandiflorum*) | A luxury oil; sedating | Good for dry skin, depression (Note: use sparingly) |
| Rose (*Rosa damascena*) | A luxury oil; sedating | Good for dry skin, depression, grief (Note: use sparingly) |
| Cedarwood (*Cedrus atlantica*) | Sedating | Good for male skincare, stress (Note: do not use in pregnancy) |
| Frankincense (*Boswellia carteri*) | Sedating, purifying | Good for mature skin, stress, mental tension |
| Patchouli (*Pogostemon cablin*) | Grounding | Good for male skincare, nervous exhaustion |

# FAQs

*How often can one have a massage?*
Every day, if you want to. Provided there are no health issues, it is a matter of choice. Regular massage works best, so try to leave it no longer than once a month.

*How do I know if I'm using the right pressure?*
Feedback from your partner is essential. Pressure is a matter of preference, so use the pressure that you feel is right, starting gently to begin with and then adjusting. The massage should be firm enough to stimulate the muscles, but if it is painful, the pressure is too hard.

*How can I be sure I'm doing it right?*
Ask your partner how the massage feels. Learning is a joint experience, and it is okay not to get it right at first. Your partner will help you. Follow the principle of massaging toward the heart and use stroking movements in between techniques to maintain the rhythm.

*The massage doesn't feel right—how do I avoid hurting my partner's feelings when telling them?*
You will not hurt your partner's feelings if you give constructive feedback. Your comments and suggestions can improve your partner's massage technique.

*How do I know if it's safe to massage?*
Check with your partner for any contraindications (see page 13). If you are in any doubt, say no and seek medical advice before continuing.

*Is massage all right when you are older?*

Massage can be very helpful for older people, whose circulation may be poorer, joints stiffer, or who may have less social contact. Do not use too much pressure. A simple hand massage can make someone feel really special.

*I haven't got time for a full massage, so how can I make it part of my day?*

Simplifying massage—or picking and choosing techniques—is fine. Work on the area that needs most attention. Even five minutes of your time can make a difference.

*I don't like following a formal routine—can I make up my own strokes?*

Massage strokes follow certain principles, and a routine provides structure to begin with. Once you have gained a little experience, it is fine to experiment. Your partner will tell you how it feels.

*I still don't feel very confident, though my partner tells me my massage feels all right. What can I do about this?*

Confidence grows with practice. But why not have a professional massage yourself, to give you some inspiration?

# Index

# Acknowledgments

## Author's acknowledgments

A huge thank you to everyone who contributed so enthusiastically to this project. Special thanks to Jessica Cowie, executive editor at Octopus, Charlotte Macey, senior editor, Penny Stock, executive art editor, and Mandy Greenfield, copy editor, for their hard work and encouragement. Thanks once again to Russell Sadur for the great photographs, photographic assistant Henry Trumble, and models Carla Collins, Olivia Garson, Fleur Roose, and Bailee Roup. Thanks also to Sarah Rade, our pregnancy model, and to Sarah Bryan and baby Georgie May Bradshaw for the baby massage.

My thanks to everyone who helped with the text, once again to W. Llewellyn McKone D.O., M.R.O., lecturer in osteopathic sports medicine, for advice on anatomy, physiology, and massage; Morgane Pairain, BSc (Hons), LicAc, MBAcC, LicTuiNa, for her contribution to the Chinese massage sequence, and to Yasuko Nomura, shiatsu practitioner, for her help with the shiatsu techniques and her arrangement of the shiatsu photos.

Finally thanks to the many teachers over the years whose ideas have inspired me and helped shape this book, especially Sara Thomas, Eve Taylor, P.J. Cousin, Dolat Pirani, Savita Patel, and Chris Jarmey.

You can contact Susan Mumford at:
www.susanmumford.co.uk

**Executive Editor:** Jessica Cowie
**Senior Editor:** Charlotte Macey
**Executive Art Editor:** Penny Stock
**Designer:** Peter Gerrish
**Photographer:** Russell Sadur
**Production Controller:** Linda Parry

**Special photography:** Octopus Publishing Group Ltd/Russell Sadur
**Other photography:**
Alamy Chris Rout 372; Image Source Black 251; ImageRite 165; Bridgeman Art Library Museo di Storia della Fotografia Fratelli Alinari, Florence 11; Getty Images Noah Clayton 384; Octopus Publishing Group 247, 385; Frazer Cunningham 327; Russell Sadur 306–309; Shutterstock Kristian Sekulic 375; Valentyn Volkov 383; Wellcome Library, London 159